Lean Six Sigma for the Medical Practice

Improving Profitability by Improving Processes

Frank Cohen, MPA, MBB
Contributing Author
Owen Dahl, MBA, FACHE, CHBC

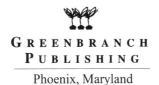

GREENBRANCH PUBLISHING

Phoenix, Maryland

PUBLISHER
Nancy Collins

EDITORIAL ASSISTANT
Jennifer Weiss

BOOK DESIGN
COVER: Jim Dodson
INTERIOR: Laura Carter
Carter Publishing Studio

COPYEDITOR
Karen Doyle

CONTENTS

ABOUT THE AUTHORS

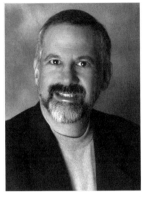

FRANK COHEN, MPA, MBB, is the senior analyst for MIT Solutions, Inc., a Clearwater, Florida-based healthcare consulting firm that specializes in process improvement and practice analytics. Frank began his extensive healthcare career as a U.S. Navy Corpsman, and he has worked as a physician assistant; medical practice administrator; researcher; hospital CEO; and, since 1988, healthcare consultant specializing in data mining, applied statistics, decision support, and process improvement. He is a certified Six Sigma Black Belt and Lean Six Sigma Master Black Belt. Over the past 20 years, he has worked on or been involved with analyzing operational, financial, and utilization issues as well as conducting compliance risk assessments for over 2000 medical practices. In addition, Frank provides litigation support services for medical practices involved in both civil and criminal actions.

Every year, Frank presents nearly 50 workshops to standing ovations of tens of thousands of healthcare professionals in every discipline and area of specialization. He is one of the most sought-after speakers in the healthcare industry with a well deserved reputation as "The Guru of Process Improvement." Recognized as an expert in critical thinking and problem solving, he is regularly engaged as both a consultant and confidante by top leaders in our industry, including CEOs, administrators, legislators, and litigators.

In addition to this and other books on medical practice analytics, Frank has participated in and published numerous articles and studies. In addition, he has trained thousands of CPAs, physicians, administrators, and others in the techniques used to improve profitability, reduce risk, increase efficiency, and improve quality of care.

His consulting experience includes hospitals, large and small medical practices, medical and professional associations, legal and accounting professionals, government agencies, and other healthcare professionals.

Frank maintains a Web site for medical practices at www.mitsi.org and for healthcare consultants at www.cpahealth.com. For information on consulting services and speaking opportunities, visit www.frankcohen.com.

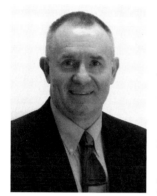

OWEN J. DAHL, MBA, FACHE, CHBC, has been active in health-care management for almost 40 years. He received his bachelor's degree from Concordia College, Moorhead, Minnesota, where he was a member of the first graduating class in the hospital administration program. He then spent more than a decade as a hospital administrator in various facilities in South Dakota. He also served in the United States Air Force.

His move to New Orleans in 1983 brought a major career change. He started a practice management and billing company, which grew to manage 65 physicians in 11 different practices with revenues well over $75 million. In 1993, he advanced to Fellow in the American College of Healthcare Executives with a paper on Total Quality Management and its application to the medical practice. He also received the distinction of becoming the first non-physician member of the Orleans Parish Medical Services Bureau Board of Directors.

Throughout his career, Owen has maintained a passion for education. He developed an adult continuing education program with Loyola University of New Orleans in physician practice management. He also is the original developer of the certification program for the Professional Association of Health Care Office Managers (PAHCOM) and the Institute of Certified Healthcare Business Consultants (ICHBC). The Institute program is currently available online through the National Society of Certified Healthcare Business Consultants (NSCHBC). He has worked with the Louisiana State University Medical School Department of Graduate Medical Education conducting seminars for students, residents, and fellows in physician practice management.

Owen is married with three children and one grandchild. He recently moved to The Woodlands, Texas. www.owendahlconsulting.com

ACKNOWLEDGMENTS

AS YOU WILL LEARN IN THE FOLLOWING PAGES, very little if any benefit comes from a vacuum, and this book is no exception. It was a team effort, and it would take another book just to thank everyone who contributed to its success. There are, however, a few folks that deserve special mention here, and it is the author's privilege and honor to take the time to do so.

Whenever I had some free time on my hands and whined about being bored, my wife, Susan, would, in a loving way, ask me how the book was coming along; and without her constant motivational talks, I would still be writing the introduction.

When I got so stuck that it was going to take the Jaws of Life to get me moving again, my friend Owen Dahl called to see what he could do to help. I asked him if he wouldn't mind writing the book for me, and as a compromise, he did agree to author the chapters on Team Building and Project Management. Friends like these are few and far between, and I owe an unrepayable debt to Owen for his help, knowledge, experience, and expertise.

My daughter Emily, after editing my third chapter of this book, called to tell me that my writing was finally getting better as a result of reading her comments and taking her advice. Without her sense of humor and commitment to her dad, I have to believe that it would have taken twice as long for the book to have been edited and produced.

My daughter Jaimee, the artist of the family, has mastered the art of photox (digital Botox), and her work on my picture for this book will eternally separate what you see there from the reality of what age has done to me.

Ron Crabtree of MetaOps, Inc., began as one of my Lean Six Sigma instructors and ended as one of my friends. In the very beginning, when I was just starting to formulate the structure of this book in my mind, Ron traveled to St. Petersburg, Florida, to spend two days with me in a small, locked room with nothing more than an easel pad and a white board. What emerged was a model for how this book was going to look.

My friend Mike Todhunter, PhD, was my Six Sigma Black Belt instructor and had a profound influence on my efforts to formulate a process improvement model that would be specific for medical practices. When the class moved into areas of manufacturing, Mike would take the time to help me understand how to apply the tools and techniques to transactional and healthcare models. Today, Mike is a mentor, and not just in the area of statistics and process improvement. His work as a spiritual leader in his community has inspired me far more than his practical knowledge and experience.

Finally, I am most grateful to Nancy Collins of Greenbranch Publishing. During the entire time that I worked on this book—from the day she agreed to publish it to when I finally delivered it more than a year behind schedule—she was my cheerleader. Many times I called her to tell her that I would understand if she wanted to tell me to forget it, but instead, she would find the right words to say that would move me forward until the next call.

In all, there are hundreds if not thousands of physicians, managers, administrators, staff, and consultants who all had a hand in this book—from their willingness to share their stories to their willingness to allow me to work with them on process improvement projects. To all of you who go unnamed, thank you very much, and I hope I will be able to return to you the value that you provided to me.

PREFACE

All happy families are the same; each unhappy family
is unhappy in its own way.
— *Anna Karenina* BY LEO TOLSTOY

All profitable practices are the same; each unprofitable
practice is unprofitable in its own way.
— *Lean Six Sigma for the Medical Practice*
BY FRANK COHEN

In the classic Clint Eastwood movie "Dirty Harry," the lead character, Detective Harry Callahan, recites one of those famous lines that cross all cultural, racial, and ethnic barriers. While holding a gun to a criminal's head, Callahan gives him the opportunity to calculate the probability that the gun has one bullet left or no bullets left. The dialogue between Harry and the perpetrator goes something like this: *"I know what you're thinking. Did he fire six shots or only five? Well, to tell you the truth, in all this excitement, I've kinda lost track myself. But being as this is a .44 Magnum, the most powerful handgun in the world, and would blow your head clean off, you've got to ask yourself one question: 'Do I feel lucky?' Well, do ya punk?"*

Having counted the number of shots fired prior to this moment, the perpetrator is not sure if Callahan fired five or six bullets but he knows it was at least five. Therefore, there is an 83.3% probability that the gun is empty (the gun holds only six bullets, so notwithstanding the binomial portion of this example, there is a one-in-six chance that the gun is not empty). The risk of being wrong, only ~17%, is relatively low; however, the consequence of being wrong is quite serious.

While not quite as dramatic as that scene, every one of us faces dozens if not hundreds of decisions every day, both in our personal and work lives. And every time we make a decision without first considering the likelihood of success or failure, we are, in essence, asking ourselves the same question. My father would tell me, "It's OK to be lucky when you're lucky." In some situations, that's OK. For others, it's simply unacceptable.

Balancing the scales are four primary factors: probability, opportunity, risk, and consequence. For example, the probability that a $500 used car will require $500 of service and repair in the next year may be quite high; say 75%. The risk may be high; however, the consequence appears low ($500). In this case, it may be OK to be lucky and it may be OK to be unlucky, even though those words poorly describe the science of our dilemma. On the other hand, a practice administrator may be tempted to over-code E/M visits for a poorly reimbursed payer and may have calculated the probability of getting caught as quite small (say, 1%). In this scenario, while the risk may be low, the consequence is very high, particularly if there are federal funds (read Medicare or Medicaid) involved. In this example, it may be OK to be lucky, but it's not OK to be unlucky.

The bottom line is this: we in the healthcare industry depend way too often on anecdote rather than evidence to make business decisions, both when the stakes are high and when they are low. We unfortunately act on the premise that if it looks like a duck and walks like a duck, it must be a duck. The truth is, the only way to tell if it is a duck is to conduct a DNA test.

The key to quality medicine is the differential diagnosis, a multivariate approach to determining what is wrong with a sick patient. It is really quite amazing to me that, in an industry that spends billions and billions of dollars on diagnostic technology that significantly reduces the guesswork for diagnosis and treatment, we still depend on "luck" for our business decisions. Imagine the following played out in the operating room. A patient is on the table, and the surgeon is about to perform a delicate procedure that requires the use of fluoroscopy. Just before the cut, the fluoroscope goes out, and the physician hesitates. He looks up at the anesthesiologist and asks her what she thinks he should do, and the anesthesiologist responds like this; "Well, doc, do you feel lucky today? Well, do you?" Even though the probability of failure may be small, the consequence is huge. Raise your hand if you would be willing to go forward if the patient's life was on the line.

"Improving Profitability by Improving Processes" is not just a concept, it's a mandate for medical providers and their staff. Even more than that, it's a moral imperative. Here's a trick question: what's the number one responsibility of a medical practice? If you said quality of care, you picked the number two responsibility. In the world according to Frank (and this is my book so for a moment, it's my world), the answer is: to be profitable. Try providing quality care to your patients with no money in the bank. Every time a practice closes (and that is happening more frequently than any of us would like), people lose their jobs, families suffer, and more importantly, the community suffers. "All profitable practices are the same" says that there is a process, a standard, if you will, that can be applied to the medical practice just as it has been for other industries (successfully, I might add) for many years. "Each unprofitable practice is unprofitable in its own way" says that without a standard business model for success, providers are held hostage to a myriad of failing strategies that, while they may have a low probability (risk) of bankrupting the practice, nonetheless have a serious potential consequence.

I have been teaching on this subject for years. In fact, I have been implementing the techniques discussed in this book for even longer. Whether you call it QI (quality improvement), SPC (statistical process control), Process Improvement, Reengineering, Six Sigma, Lean, Kaizen, or whatever, the bottom line is this: unless we (the provider industry) begin to embrace integration of successful business models into our practices, we are bound to incur failure at a higher rate than is necessary. Here's another trick question: what's the primary responsibility of a payer? To be profitable. OK, not such a trick question after all. Saving the melodrama, the fact is, we are in a war with a sophisticated enemy (payers) that has been employing advanced business techniques for many years, and it's time we, the provider side, started fighting back. So, let me ask you a question: Do you feel lucky today? Well, do you?

Introduction

IN NOVEMBER 1999, the Institute of Medicine released a report concluding that nearly 98,000 deaths in America were the result of medical mistakes and could have been prevented. This began a rush toward excellence within our industry in order to identify the causes of and find solutions to what this report described as a huge failure of our healthcare system. The report set as its goal a 50% reduction in errors over the following five years. Zoom to April 8, 2008, and a study conducted by HealthGrades, a controversial company that creates and reports grades, if you will, for hospitals, physicians, nursing homes, and other healthcare facilities. The HealthGrades report concluded that medical errors, in all forms, resulted in 238,337 preventable deaths between 2004 and 2008 with an associated cost of around $8.8 billion. And the feeding frenzy continues . . .

In any segment of society, there are those that seem to take advantage of the weaknesses of others, and the situation described above is no exception with respect to the diversion it created within our industry. While so much effort was focused on the movement to improve quality and reduce medical errors (don't get me wrong, a worthy and necessary endeavor), there were those that used this as a diversionary tactic to shift the focus to the dollars measured as a percentage of our gross domestic product from the actual issue of what was being spent on healthcare.

Today, we find ourselves in a different sort of healthcare crisis, and it appears to be the medical providers—the physicians—that are the target of these attacks. Make no mistake; we are at war, and the stakes are high. We can't measure the losses only in dollars but in the human lives that are affected, not by medical mistakes but rather by jobs and stress. And it's not through poor quality but rather as a result of shady practices, ignorance, mismanagement, and a gross disregard for business principles and processes.

1

I am no stranger to the quality problems we face in our country as it pertains to the practice of medicine. Many simply don't consider the enormous complexity of the human body and its systems. And there is a perception among the public that the doctors' role is to fix what we break through poor health practices. That unrealistic expectation drives much of the angst that many researchers express in their studies. This book, however, is not about ways to improve the quality of medical care in America, or even more overwhelming, on a global scale. I know that there are tools at our disposal that can measure and affect quality of care but I am a believer that, within the universe of the medical practice, quality of care is more of a cultural issue than a malleable process. This book is based on one of two premises: that there is a baseline of quality that meets or exceeds what is acceptable; or, as some may believe, we just ignore that idea completely. In either case, by removing the burden of clinical quality from these pages, we are free to focus solely on the business at hand; which is, frankly, just the business at hand.

I am grateful for those that have preceded me with regard to exploring the use of process improvement tools employed by other industries for many years and applying them to healthcare. We should not be a stranger to the struggles that others have faced. This type of ignorance perpetuates our problems and makes us feel like victims. We are, in fact, volunteers, and the idea is to either improve our surroundings or to find somewhere else to play. Improvement, whether couched in the form of formal process improvement or personal improvement, needs to be continuous, and this requires courage, commitment, and resources. Lacking any of these will normally guarantee failure. These three criteria are both internal and external, and under most circumstances, require a team effort. In America, nearly 80% of medical practices are defined as small practices, with three or fewer physicians. And having worked in that environment, I know that the concept of "team building" can seem like a joke. In a solo practice, you are the team—the process owner, the champion, the stakeholder, and all the other positions contained within the lexicon of the formalized models that follow. Still, there is opportunity to be involved as a team member, small and insignificant as that may seem.

This book is surrounded by and invested in the tools and applications of Lean Six Sigma. Technically speaking, Lean Six Sigma is an amalgamation of Six Sigma and Lean, each one a unique model with its own set of tools. Six Sigma was born within the manufacturing industry; and to this day, it is still identified by that realm. Six Sigma is optimized for businesses involved in the manufacturing sector. Lean, while more adaptable to the service industry, still has its roots in manufacturing. Even from the standpoint of transactional businesses—businesses that are more vested in the service side of the market—Lean and Six Sigma need, at times, significant modifications to be of value to the whole of a medical practice. Still, medical practices are idiosyncratic in their own way; and therefore, I have developed what we call Total Practice Improvement, or TPI. Lean Six Sigma combines the tools and techniques of Lean and Six Sigma, as the name suggests. TPI takes those tools and techniques and culls the ones that are not applicable to the specific needs of the practice and eliminates them from the lexicon. It's quite interesting, actually; if we are going to work toward maximum efficiency, it would seem that the model we use should be efficient as well.

In Chapter 1 (WIIFM, or What's In It For Me), I talk about the different reasons that different groups of professionals might find value in this book. The fact is, it's not for everyone. And of those who find reason and purpose within these pages, not everyone will have success in implementing the benefits. Not all projects are candidates for these concepts, and more often, the practice does not have a culture of improvement. For the latter, read on, and you will find hope in the suggestions we make here to get buy-in from owners and upper management.

Chapter 2 (Why Process Improvement?) introduces the concept of process improvement and even more important, defines what is a process and how it applies to every business, not just the medical practice. In this chapter, we will look at not only the differences between process improvement and other models, such as reengineering, but also the similarities. I haven't invented something here; only identified an efficient delivery system and incorporated it into what it is we do—practice medicine.

Chapter 3 (Team Building) was written by my good friend Owen Dahl and discusses the methods that are often employed to create and maintain working teams. More specifically, we will focus on process improvement teams and how they differ from some of the other types of teams we often encounter. In this chapter, we will address the different roles that team members play and more importantly, the necessity of each team member to define and understand his or her responsibilities. Teams are not always easy to create but once they get up and running (correctly), they are a *force majeure* within the organization. You can also expect to spend some time learning about the four basic stages of team development: forming, storming, norming, and performing, and what to do to lessen the negative and improve the positive aspects of each of these stages.

Chapter 4 (Project Management) was also written by Owen, which is very fortuitous as he is perhaps the most preeminently qualified person I have met when it comes to this topic. At first glance, this chapter may feel a bit diversionary, but it has an important position within the process improvement arena. Oftentimes, newcomers to process improvement see selecting the project as a no-brainer. And more often than not, this leads to wasted resources when, later down the road, they discover that they picked the wrong project or an inappropriate project. Further, being able to manage the project through to completion is almost a science unto itself. Project management can be a huge topic when applied to general projects; yet when it is focused on the area of continuous process improvement projects, it promotes a manageable and efficient process. Many organizations attempt to begin process improvement projects without having a management manifesto in place. And while the project may, in fact, succeed, it will often fall apart shortly after implementation due to a lack of considerations, such as risk analysis, control management, and other components that, left out, add a degree of porosity to the improvement results.

Chapter 5 (The TPI Toolbox) is a bit more complex in the information presented as it deals with the specific tools that are necessary to get the job done. All told, I narrowed the field from over 60 tools to just 20, not just for the purpose of manageability but because so many of the others are focused on other industrial areas, such as manufacturing, financial, or retail. And while there is a bit of cross-functionality for tools in all industries, there is no getting away from the anomalies found within the business of the medical practice. Here, we begin with a discussion of the concept of a process improvement toolbox with special focus on those that are foundational to all improvement activities, such as process and value stream mapping, voice of the customer, critical to quality trees, Takt time, load balancing, and many others. For each tool listed, specific examples are given to elucidate the application of that tool within the medical practice.

Chapter 6 (Deployment Platforms) goes deep into the application of the tools within a deployment platform. Platforms come in different sizes and models as do medical practices; and here, I try to link up one with the other. We will spend quite a bit of time studying the DMAIC (Define, Measure, Analyze, Improve, Control) platform as this is the king. If you can get your head around this, the others will fall right into their proper place, giving you the ability to pick and choose based on your specific needs. This is a chapter about model building—about developing a consistent and polymorphic way to incorporate solutions and change within a consistent and understandable framework. Expect to also spend a bit of time with PDSA (Plan, Do, Study, and Act) as this is becoming the most popular platform for small to medium-size practices. In fact, some certifying organizations are requiring that physicians complete a PDSA project in order to become recertified in their specialty.

In Chapter 7 (What's Next), I will close with a bit of philosophizing, so let me apologize in advance. We are, as I complete of this manuscript, facing perhaps the most challenging time in the history of medicine. Physician practices are facing financial problems that very few ever believed would be a part of their business model. Practices are being purchased, sold, traded, and pushed in and out of markets like a tradable commodity, which, to many, they have become. In this chapter, I will prognosticate (only, however, a little) about our future with and without process improvement. And as you can likely guess, the latter looks quite bleak.

As you proceed, remember that this is a journey and not a destination. Projects will start, and they will finish. Some will be successful, and some will not. Some of you will find that it is all but impossible to implement process improvement within your organization, while others will be cranking out solutions and improvements after reading only the first few chapters. Heck, some of you probably know more about this than I do and have stories to tell that would motivate the most skeptical of the bunch.

This is a journey specifically because of the need to be continuous. Once a project is closed, successful or not, it is usually time to begin the next, and when that is complete . . . well, you get the point. Don't forget: quality is expensive, and process improvement is likely the most effective and efficient tool to keep the practice in a position to provide quality care—our number two responsibility!

ONE

WIIFM
(What's In It for Me)

IRRESPECTIVE OF THE TREMENDOUS VALUE of the material that follows, and disregarding the brilliant use of prose and the English language, and even ignoring the elegant transitions between paragraphs, no one will finish this book unless they find within a specific benefit to themselves. More specifically, you probably won't read much past this chapter unless you have a good understanding of what's in it for you (WIIFY?). I accept this and am willing to admit that I am the same way. Whether it is a book on statistics or another John Grisham novel, unless I feel that there is something of benefit for me, I won't take the time and energy to read it.

The truth is (and I already know this), everyone will find some benefit to this book. Even those who are not in the healthcare field, if they read carefully and visualize the use of the tools for whatever industry in which they are engaged, will find some benefit in the pages that follow. But this book was not written for them; it was written for those that labor within the healthcare industry. Healthcare, while ultimately no more or less a business than, say, a dry cleaning establishment, is unique in the way that every other business in every other industry is unique.

We deal in human lives not machines, yet the way that we measure outcomes is virtually the same. Ours is an industry of uncertainty and continuous growth in learning about complex systems, yet the tools we use to measure success or failure of our model are virtually the same. Each practice, irrespective of specialty and location, is both similar and different at the same time. We are an industry that deals in high risk and two extreme outcome potentials. Success is celebrated through the continuity of a quality life, while failure is catastrophic not only to the patient but his or her family and the provider as well. While Six Sigma as a measurement of success is touted in the manufacturing sector as a badge of honor, in healthcare, achieving a level of quality measured the same way would result in the unnecessary deaths of tens of thousands of patients a year. Ours is an industry of higher criticality and a much higher standard of quality than any other industry out there, except, perhaps, the airline industry.

Continuous Practice Improvement is not an original thought but rather a transmorphic concept that presents the case for a commitment to improving the overall efficiency of a medical practice (although this is just as applicable to other organizations, such as hospitals, nursing homes, etc.). Where many people get confused is the link between efficiency and quality, and how these two critical areas of business link is a fair and necessary question. As discussed, we might ask the following question: "What is the primary responsibility of a medical practice?" and most respond with, "Providing high quality care to patients." Notwithstanding the Hippocratic oath, this is, in nearly any situation, unachievable without a primary goal of profitability. Think about it; quality is expensive—quality staff, quality equipment, quality supplies, quality, quality, quality. Without revenue, and more specifically without revenue in excess of expenses (profit), quality is mostly unaffordable. Now granted, we do see situations in which a healthcare organization may be deficit-funded through a trust or government subsidy, but these are few and far between and in any case, still depend on a form of efficiency within the organization.

So let's try to define the WIIFM for those of you that have taken the time to read this far. Whether you are a physician or allied healthcare provider, an administrator, front-line staffer, an individual responsible for funding, a regulator, or even a consultant, there is something in it for you.

THE HEALTHCARE PROVIDER

I went to college to study pre-med with the goal of becoming a doctor. A stint in the Navy interrupted that goal but didn't change my direction; and four years after entering the service, I was discharged as a physician's assistant. I spent the next eight years in clinical practice and took from that experience two great lessons. The first is that the general public simply has no idea of the level of difficulty involved in both becoming a physician and working as a physician. The second is the enormous amount of stress that most physicians experience day to day. That was 30 years ago, and it has only gotten worse since then. Back then, we saw a patient, submitted a claim, and got paid. The fact is, now is not the best of times to be a physician, yet there are those that continue to commit their lives to what we in the industry have come to understand as a heroic pursuit.

The physician of today no longer has the luxury of just practicing medicine. Today's physician needs to understand the basics of compliance, law, personnel management, coding, billing, etc. The physician of today assumes the role of manager and CEO whether he or she likes it or not. Many physicians who were in private practice have elected the option of going from small business owner to employee in order to avoid many of the hassles and stresses of owning a medical practice. Very few are going from employee to business owner, and those that do don't necessarily stay there for long.

Recently, the American Medical Association released the results of a year-long study called the National Health Insurer Report Card, which identified a significant level of ambiguity and inefficiency within the claims process.[1] While much of the study's focus was on the payers, it was also clear that physician offices play a key role in ensuring that claims are submitted accurately and timely if they expect to be paid accurately and in a timely manner. In fact, if any other business ran with the level of inefficiency of most medical practices, they would be, well, out of business. Like it or not, particularly in the private practice sector, the physician owner is the CEO of the business, and knowing and understanding the basics of how to run an efficient business is key to success. Even in the presence of the most capable staff, it is always the owner that takes the hit when revenues are down or a compliance audit goes south.

This book is for the physician provider, and if you take the time to read it and practice what is preached, you will have a more successful and profitable business.

ADMINISTRATOR

Now here's a job that many people would eschew. Not because it isn't important but because it is one of the toughest jobs anyone can have right now. By last count, the Internal Revenue Code and Regulations contained 9097 pages. The Code of Federal Regulations is 16,845 pages and contains around three million words. Between the *Medicare Carriers Manual*, updates and transmittals, E/M coding guidelines, compliance rules and regulations, Stark legislation, National Correct Coding Initiative technical specifications, etc., healthcare beats them all!. The typical managed care contract has gone from 4 pages to 80 pages, and even many of our seasoned healthcare attorneys are taxed to make sense of the whole picture.

With reference to the National Health Insurer Report Card mentioned above, the results of the 15 metrics chosen for the study painted a grim picture of the business state of our claims process, the heart and soul of what drives practice profitability.[1] The study focused on seven national payers along with Medicare. The sad news was that Medicare, with respect to efficiency, accuracy, timeliness, clarity, transparency, and in nearly every other category, came out the winner; and second place was a long distance from there. Imagine this: you get paid twice a month based on your employment agreement, let's say the first and fifteenth of each month. How long would you continue with your job if you had to spend up to 14% of your paycheck on making sure that you got paid on time and got paid what you were supposed to get paid? Probably not very long but that is what a physician faces every day. But wait, not really what the physician faces but rather what you, the administrator, faces.

I have worked as a practice administrator, and I know how the hierarchal structure works against us; blame rolls downhill. We, in turn, can take it to our billing managers (if we have any), our contract specialist (if we have one), or the coder (if we have one) but ultimately, we hold the hot potato. In a small practice, it is the administrator that pretty much takes on all of those jobs and is held accountable for what amounts to problems that simply feel out of his or her control. In a larger practice, while there are more people to blame, the result is the same. The buck (or the lack of a buck) stops here!

This book provides the administrator with a toolbox that not only works to solve the problem of payer inefficiency, but helps the practice to achieve near 100% efficiency by analyzing, understanding, and improving business processes so at least, from your perspective, you have done as much as you can to maximize revenue and minimize expense. After all, that is the definition of profitability. If you really take the time to study this book and to use the tools given here, you will be nothing short of a hero in the eyes of your doctors. Who should read this book? A lot of folks, and you, the administrator, are one of those that will surely benefit from what is to follow.

FRONT-LINE STAFF

Some may think that I am lazy for grouping everyone short of the doc and the administrator into this category, but that just isn't the case. From a traditional standpoint, some folks in this category may have a more important role, or a harder job, or more responsibility, and even assume more risk. I spent several years as a Navy corpsman, and I learned that while the officers got the glory and the benefits, it was the non-commissioned officers (NCOs) that contributed the most to the success or failure of any operation. I would take a chief petty officer over a captain any day, and any petty officer over a commissioned officer that same day. Why? Because it was us "grunts" that did the real work. And it is the front-line staffers that carry out the steps and functions that determine a practice's ultimate success or failure.

Every employee of every organization has an important role to play with respect to process improvement and efficiency of operations. Not every employee, however, is motivated to that point. I have always been a strong believer that every employee within the medical practice should share in the bonus plan because every employee can make a difference when it comes to profitability. Unfortunately, not all (or even very many) practices have caught on to that yet. Those that do have realized a significant improvement in overall quality of care, staff morale, patient satisfaction, and overall efficiency, and, as a result, increased profitability. But let's not be surprised that this approach hasn't caught on more widely. There are those who feel that it takes up to 15 years for positive medical discoveries to even make it to the practice.

If you have a strong work ethic and really want to be involved in seeing your organization grow and prosper, then this is the book for you. This book was not written as a reference book to sit on a shelf somewhere; rather, read it and use the tools, and you will be richly rewarded for your efforts.

THE CONSULTANT

While fishing one day with an old high school buddy who had become a physician, the discussion got around to the value of consultants. Being a healthcare consultant talking to a physician, I was very interested in his take on this because selling consulting services to physicians is always a challenge. To explain his position, my friend took off his watch and held it up and said, "Hiring a consultant is like paying someone else to tell me what time it is." Ouch!

"The first thing I look for when I consider a consultant," he told me, "is someone who knows more than I do about the issue." Not a bad perspective, really, when you consider how easy it is to call yourself a consultant. I have been a healthcare consultant since 1988, and my most important and pressing of goals is to be at the leading edge, if not leading the edge, with respect to business innovation. He had a great point; why would any of us hire someone to handle an issue if we know more about it than the consultant does? Here's a better question: what new things have you learned in the past year or two? I spend as much time reading journal articles and books and attending conferences as I do actually consulting. The reason is simple: if I don't, then I'm just like every other consultant out there, and that substantially increases my competition and decreases my value. Personally, I do a lot of things that other healthcare consultants don't do and that decreases my competition and increases my value.

So what new things have you learned this year that your competitors have not? If you have been following any of the current literature, you would see that process improvement, and more specifically the use of Lean and Six Sigma, is moving headlong into healthcare—and not just into hospitals but medical practices as well. There is a movement afoot to bring these techniques directly to physicians, and the good news is physicians are responding.

If you are a consultant and you want to broaden your scope, increase the value of your services, and knock your competition into the cheap seats, then this is the book for you.

THE PAYER

Even writing the heading gives me the chills. The payer is the classic enemy of the medical practice, and it just doesn't have to be that way. This natural enmity has evolved over the past 20 years, and somehow, we all accept it as standard operating procedure. It's like having a military base in Cuba; some things just don't make sense. When I was in practice, things were a lot more congenial, and the payers were our friends. See a patient, submit a claim, and get paid. In the National Health Insurer Report Card, it was pretty evident that the percentage of claims that gets paid accurately the first time around is well below any reasonable standard. But what the report card doesn't say is who is at fault. Now we can take some license and say that because Medicare is up there and under HIPAA and pretty much all claims are filed the same way, the private payers should also be, well, up there when it comes to paying on time and accurately. And while the practice shares in its part of the blame, the payers, if they chose to tighten things up, could have a substantial impact on the overall efficiency of the claims process. In essence, there are about 40 companies that control around 80% of all the claims paid to around 750,000 physicians. Now who do you think is in the best position to effect a positive change?

If you are a payer and considering whether you should read this book, think about the overall savings that would be realized by your organization as well as the physicians. Every time a physician appeals a denied claim or has to track a late or missing claim, it costs the payer time, resources, and money just is it does the practice. Lack of transparency with regard to fee schedules and ambiguity in other areas require more work than is necessary in what should be a more open architecture. If I were in charge, I would want to run as efficiently and transparently as possible, reduce my costs as much as I could, charge premiums that reflect a fair market value, and still make a killing with regard to profit. If you share this goal with me and you are a payer, then read on! This is definitely the book for you.

FINANCIAL PROFESSIONALS

The nature and picture of the business of healthcare are, as mentioned above, experiencing a very dynamic metamorphosis. And one area that is changing the fastest has to do with the financial and operational aspect of the medical practice; specifically, merging of smaller local practices into larger regional groups, and the renewed interest by hospitals in purchasing (or creating) physician practices. At the same time, we see declines in reimbursement and legislation that works against this type of business model.

Smart financial professionals always engage in a feasibility study to determine the likelihood of success (or failure) of a new venture, and an often overlooked component of this type of study is the true potential of the venture. Think about it; we look at the market (prevalence and preponderance), reimbursement trends, technological advancements, patient volume, operational capacity, etc. in order to determine where a group is *now*, but how about where a group *could be*? I have been involved in many of these types of analyses, and I can tell you that knowing the capability of a venture is more important than understanding its current state. What about a practice (or a bunch of practices) that are underperforming? What about potential compliance risks? How about we create a "what-if" scenario based on the potential of an organization to perform if it were more efficient?

Throughout this book, we discuss, sometimes in great detail, ways in which assessments of efficiency can be conducted to provide a better look at the potential of a business venture rather than accepting the current state as the best state. If you are involved in financing these types of ventures or if you are going to be the recipient of this kind of change, you should definitely read this book first. Your overall success may depend on it!

REGULATORS

As we move into a period of political turmoil regarding healthcare policy, regulators have stressed the need to do two things simultaneously: make sure everyone has access to healthcare and do so in such a way as to control the expense of such an open model. This is quite a challenge, particularly considering the way that healthcare is currently managed. Few would disagree that our healthcare system is broken with respect to the business model while most would agree that medical technology in the United States is at the top of the list. This naturally introduces what amounts to a very delicate balance between quality, access, and costs; not an undertaking for the meek or weak-hearted.

As a result, a heated debate has surfaced over whether the system should be fixed (a bandage approach) or overhauled (a reengineering approach). All sides have presented data and statistics to support their respective positions, yet there hasn't surfaced a comprehensive analysis that deals specifically with the facts without a political bias. Which is sad, as that is what is needed to drill down to a real solution.

Gray areas exist in all camps but if the true goal is to reach some sort of equilibrium regarding the three criteria (access, quality, and cost), it would behoove those in a position to effect change to take a look at how the process improvement concepts presented in this book could help. If you are a regulator and your motives are really to find the most effective way to create and maintain the best healthcare system in the world, then this book is also for you.

Reference

1. American Medical Association. National Health Insurer Report Card. 2009; www.ama-assn.org/ama1/pub/upload/mm/368/2009-nhirc-long.pdf.

TWO

Why Process Improvement?

A FTER WORLD WAR II, growth in healthcare was tremendous. Increasing profits only meant increasing fees. Newly formed health insurance companies paid the entire healthcare bill. Most patients never had to reach into their pockets to cover the cost of their healthcare. Technology was increasing at an amazing rate. X-rays, imaging, ultrasound, surgical techniques, heart-lung machines, pacemakers, and all of the technological techniques and devices that promised to deliver almost immortality drove the industry. No other country could touch it. America was the place to be for healthcare. For 30 years plus, we enjoyed the benefits of an immature market and of unprecedented growth and open-ended profit potential. Every mother wanted her son to be a physician, and medical schools popped up all over the country to accommodate the demand.

The industry began to mature in the 1980s. Technology was getting out of control with respect to costs incurred in R&D, which eventually translated into fees for the consumer. The consumers themselves changed from the patient to the corporation as more companies chose to be self-insured. Alternative payer systems emerged, like HMOs, PPOs, MSOs, IPAs, and dozens of other managed care plans. Some made it, others didn't. But all were focused on lowering the cost of the healthcare delivery system. One problem was that while private industry realized the need to move ahead with cost-reduction systems, the medical practice did not. Because of years of a boom market and enormous financial growth, physicians ignored the warnings. There was no sense of urgency so they were slow to recognize what was coming down the pike.

The shakeout began in the 1990s. Many of the managed care organization plans were not only very successful, but surprised many industry analysts. They were raking in hundreds of millions of dollars in profits while physicians' income was on the decline. They had figured out how to deliver services, control costs, increase efficiency, and generate huge profits through the use of process technology.

Unfortunately, the physician was not the only one to suffer. Because most of the major players and payers had very little interest in the quality of care delivered to the patient, everyone but the payers stood to lose. Patients were denied necessary treatments because they did not pass the test of value, price, and positive outcome designed by the payers. Information abounded, more than ever before, but the payers were reluctant to share it with the physicians. It was a one-way-communication street. On the other hand, physicians were feeling forced to figure out how to beat the system and as a result were helping to shape laws and regulations to the benefit of the payers. In essence, it all hit the fan.

What does the future look like? Inefficient, low-quality practices will disappear. This reduces the number of competitors and helps stabilize the market. This leads to healthy competition and reduces the criticality of the current crunch. Those medical practices prepared to move forward with the business technologies necessary to improve efficiency, quality, and profitability will be those that survive and even prosper after the shakeout is over. Those that hang on to tradition, old ways of doing business, and their money with a vengeance will disappear. In any mature market, the strong (and the smart) are the survivors. All that is required to make it is a commitment to change. That's it. And what is it that needs to change for most practices? Only everything, that's all.

In this chapter, we are going to take some time to get better acquainted with not only the concept of a process, but also just what we mean when we talk about process improvement. It wasn't too long ago that strategic planning was a chic phrase that was being promoted to medical practices. Strategic planning, as it was, was profitable for consultants and facilitators for a number of different reasons. Certainly, billable hours or a project fee was one area but the biggest was that very few practices, if any, were able to substantiate the benefits and/or success rate of these plans. Most of the so-called strategic plans that I have reviewed over the years lacked any kind of formal process for evaluating metrics that are normally used to determine success or failure. Hey, if you were conducting strategic planning sessions for docs, you just couldn't lose. Notice how the fire went out and very few practices were getting engaged in this type of activity more recently? That's because, with some exceptions, either the strategic plan produced little or no value or, if it did, there was no way to tell.

Virtually every business is in business to provide a high-quality product or service to its customers and in doing so, generate at least enough revenue to stay in business, and more often, to make a profit for the owners and/or stockholders. As such, virtually every business, whether large or small, whether engaged in manufacturing or service, whether serving the general public or a vertical market, is run around processes. Process improvement is a natural event that simply seeks to take those processes and make them as efficient as possible. In essence, process improvement simply means making things better. It's not about putting out fires or finding a quick fix to a problem but rather a cultural approach to finding out what is wrong and what it will take to improve the bottom li

WHA

A process, in its most basic state, is   ken in order to accomplish something. A pro   rning and getting ready for work or as compl   ing electricity at a nuclear power plant. Pro   atient or performing an MRI or x-ray. Condu   nt to the hospital, and even disposing of bio-l   s.

If we were to examine a simple pi   ld find that there are many steps and decisic   en you wake up, you have to decide if it is a w   er you are going to get up or not. Other deci   ing to wear (maybe based on the weather or   ˷ (based on if you are hungry or not and if you even   ꞇ), what route to take to work (maybe dependent on the time of day and traffic patterns), etc. For each of these decision points, there are steps involved. For example, if you choose to eat breakfast, steps may include getting a griddle, heating it on the stove, preparing a couple of eggs the way you like them, getting out any condiments, and when finished, washing and putting away the items used to make breakfast. While we don't always pay attention to these steps in a formalized way, they do, in fact, build a process, and whether or not we are successful in implementing that process (or any process) is dependent on our approach.

THE PROCESS OF PROCESS IMPROVEMENT

Having defined the "what" of a process, it is important to understand the overall effect a good or a bad process can have on a business. As stated above, it is reasonable to expect that, for almost all businesses, providing a quality product or service while making a profit is a primary goal. Healthcare is no different in that quality and profitability go hand in hand in order to define success. Process improvement benefits the organization because it provides a model to improve the quality and profitability of what we do in a structured, ordered, and measurable way. I have worked with many practices that have resorted to knee-jerk reactions to problems, thinking that they were engaging in process improvement but instead were using anecdotal (non-data oriented) thinking, relying instead on gut instinct and/or advice from other people for their decisions. Now I want to say here that I am not an opponent of instinct or experiential actions, but these are most effective when combined with more formal data analyses and process improvement activities. I have seen practices that, due to increasing accounts receivables times and/or decreases in collections, decided to outsource their billing function to a billing company only to realize that this created collateral damage that was not anticipated, such as excess full-time equivalents needed to monitor the billing company and correct its mistakes, inadequate monitoring or reporting by the billing company, and other administrative issues. Had they taken the time to map the processes involved in the revenue cycle—to analyze the steps within each process—they may have found other alternatives that would have been more effective or at the least, been prepared with a contingency plan for negative effects of their decision. In some cases, reactionary decisions work but this takes us back to the "It's OK to be lucky when you are lucky" model.

Process improvement, as defined here, is a focus on improving the steps and decisions that are involved in each of the processes identified by the organization. This brings us to another concept in our process improvement model and that is the idea of continuous process improvement. So often, an organization will engage in process improvement as a tool; but rather than seeing it as a standard business approach, the organization sees it as a one-time event designed to fix a one-time problem. This is so counterproductive that, at times, it is worse than doing nothing at all. In nearly every process improvement event that I have witnessed, there have been collateral effects that, pointing to relationships between steps or processes, needed to be addressed. But because there was no advanced thought about a continuous model, they were not addressed.

Continuous process improvement, then, is the archetypical goal of this book. Depending on what source you consult, businesses should commit between 4% and 11% of their resources to continuous process improvement. Instead of running 20 years behind most businesses, medical practices should be in the front of the pack. Continuous process improvement, while not the sole solution to what ails us, is one of the most critical and well-proven examples that we have to follow.

PROCESS IMPROVEMENT VS. REENGINEERING

Michael Hammer, considered to be the father of reengineering, defines it as "the fundamental rethinking and radical redesign of business processes to achieve dramatic improvements in critical, contemporary measures of performance, such as cost, quality, service and speed."[1]

Reengineering is, in effect, starting over. It is not about fixing problems, putting bandages on small inefficiencies, changing a few policies or procedures, or hiring or firing staff. Reengineering, while it may incorporate all of the above, entails much more. In reengineering, tradition means nothing. In thinking about the process of reengineering, there is one critical question to ask: "If I had to do the whole thing over, knowing then what I know now, how would I design this business?" The most important point to remember is that reengineering calls for radical changes—radical in the sense that they are major and swift and challenge our understanding of how things should be.

Process improvement differs from reengineering in that, more often than not, improvements can be made incrementally, quickly, and with minimal use of resources. Certainly this is not always the case, but we see it enough times to build our confidence that reengineering is a worst-case scenario. Often even when we see the need to reengineer, process improvement tools and techniques both precede and are integrated into the model. Reengineering is often disruptive and destructive and requires enterprise-wide commitment and sacrifice. While process improvement projects can sometimes feel this way, using deployment platforms such as PDSA, Deming Wheel, or Kaizen Events often produces benefits far in excess of the necessary resources.

UNDERSTANDING EFFICIENCY

Efficiency is the ability to deliver the highest quality product or service in the least amount of time for the lowest possible cost. It defines a process of functional tasks that are used to produce the product or service, also known as the cycle. For example, an efficient light bulb delivers the greatest amount of light using the least amount of electricity while giving off the least amount of heat.

Today's typical medical practice, as it has evolved, has become the antithesis of efficiency because of multiple levels of management, decision-making processes, defensive practices, job specialization, and the lack of patient feedback.

In his book *Reengineering the Medical Practice*, Jon A. Hultman, MD, uses the example of Christmas lights to define this problem.[2] In a serial lighting string, if one light burns out, the entire string of lights fails to work. It becomes necessary to replace each bulb, one at a time, to find the bad one. If there are two bad bulbs, the task becomes daunting at best, and if there are more bad bulbs, the process of fixing the light string becomes impossible. Even more important, to fix the light string requires more expenditure in time and total resources than it would take to buy a new set of lights. Another problem is that even if you were to find the bad bulbs, you may have to replace, or "fix," many bulbs that are working fine.

In a parallel string of lights, only the bulbs that are bad fail to light. Not only does this make it more efficient to locate and replace these bad bulbs, but it still allows the string of lights to function until the replacements are made.

The typical medical practice starts with two or three employees. At first, they can perform each other's jobs. As the practice grows and more employees are added, they begin to specialize. This process of task specialization increases the problems of efficiency. During peak times, bottlenecks occur. During absenteeism, sometimes the entire function ceases completely, interrupting the entire business cycle.

In this way, the typical medical practice is like the serial string of lights. There may be several tasks within a process and processes within a cycle that are "bad," so to speak. Not only are these difficult to locate, but in the end, it may require fewer total resources to completely redo a process than it does to try to locate, identify, and fix the bad areas.

Another example of inefficiency can be illustrated by looking at the design of a highway. Let's assume a highway has three lanes in either direction for 30 miles. At some point, after traffic flow has reached a peak of 45,000 vehicles per hour, there is construction that reduces flow to two lanes for several miles. At two lanes of traffic, the maximum flow is 30,000 vehicles per hour.

Several problems occur as a result of the construction area. There is less room for the same volume of traffic. If one-third of the cars must merge into the other two lanes, each of the cars in the other two lanes must slow down to allow room for the merging vehicle. This requires a longer traffic line as the width is being reduced. Let's say that each vehicle must slow down for 10 seconds to adjust to the change in traffic flow. If there are 500 cars slowing down during the three-mile construction zone, this accounts for 50 minutes of delay time for the 501st car.

This time variation per vehicle is cumulative and referred to as a statistical variance. These statistical variances are difficult to predict and even more difficult to control. The only solutions to this problem would be to either reduce the amount of traffic allowed on the highway or to widen the road back to three lanes through the construction zone. If you decrease the number of vehicles allowed to enter the highway, you would create bottlenecks on the entrance ramps and roads leading to them. If you widen the highway to four lanes prior to the construction, you only decrease the time it takes to get to the bottleneck and increase the statistical variance from merging four lanes into two lanes. In this example, fixing anything except the cause of the problem consumes resources and does not increase efficiency or quality.

In a medical practice, a bottleneck may occur at the point of collecting the fee for the service. When the patient has completed the visit and is returned to the front desk, the patient may not know that he or she is expected to pay at the time of visit. Maybe the patient's insurance status has not yet been verified, and his or her payment responsibility is not clear. This causes confusion and a slow down (statistical variance), which then backs up other patients waiting to see the doctor, pay their bill, or schedule a return appointment. If another staff member breaks away from what he or she is doing to help, the tasks for which that staffer is responsible get behind, and this causes other bottlenecks.

In this example, the bottleneck could be eliminated if the patient was sent information forms in advance to be completed prior to the first appointment. Then insurance can be verified, including deductibles and patient co-insurance, ahead of time. The patient would know what to expect with respect to the approximate cost of the visit and what payment methods are accepted.

THE SEVEN PHASES OF CHANGE

If you ask most people how they feel about change, most would likely associate it negatively, even if their past experiences with change have been, for the most part, positive. The idea of change conjures up feelings of anxiety, fear, insecurity, stress, and uncertainty. My friend Henry's favorite saying was, "If the only thing consistent in our lives is change, then how come we never get used to it?"

Change is such an important and common event within companies that many have people whose sole responsibility is change management. And change management is often times a discipline defined more by psychology than by business acumen. Change is, in fact, like most everything else discussed in this book, a process. And like every other process, it involves a series of steps that are necessary to reach a successful conclusion.

It's quite interesting, actually, that the steps (or phases) associated with the change process are not wholly dissimilar to the five phases of death. In fact, to many workers I have spoken with over the years, the latter would be preferable to the fear encountered by the threat of change.

In his article on the change process, Oliver Recklies identified seven distinct phases by which people perceive change.[3]

- **Phase 1—Shock and Surprise:** Confrontation with unexpected situations can happen "by accident" (e.g., losses in particular business units) or through planned even⸱ workshops for personal development and team performance impro⸱ uations make people realize that their own patterns of doing thi⸱ the new conditions. Thus, their own perceived competence d⸱

- **Phase 2—Denial and Refusal:** People activate values as support for their conviction that change is not necessary. Hence, they believe there is no need for change; their perceived competency increases again.
- **Phase 3—Rational Understanding:** People realize the need for change. According to this insight, their perceived competence decreases again. People focus on finding short-term solutions, thus they cure only the symptoms. There is no willingness to change their own patterns of behavior.
- **Phase 4—Emotional Acceptance:** This phase, which is also called "crisis," is the most important one. Only if management succeeds in creating a willingness for changing values, beliefs, and behaviors, will the organization be able to exploit its real potential. In the worst case, however, change processes will be stopped or slowed down here.
- **Phase 5—Exercising and Learning:** The new acceptance of change creates a new willingness for learning. People start to try new behaviors and processes. They will experience success and failure during this phase. It is the change managers use to create some early wins (e.g., by starting with easier projects). This will lead to an increase in peoples' own perceived competence.
- **Phase 6—Realization:** People gather more information by learning and exercising. This knowledge has a feedback effect. People understand which behavior is effective in which situation. This, in turn, opens up their minds for new experiences. These extended patterns of behavior increase organizational flexibility. Perceived competency reaches a higher level than prior to the change.
- **Phase 7—Integration:** People totally integrate their newly acquired patterns of thinking and acting. The new behaviors become routine.

Willingness on the part of management to embrace both the change itself as well as the emotional manifestation that change creates is what is necessary to ensure transitional events with the least amount of resistance. After all, as Henry would say, "The pain is not in the change; it's in the resistance."

IF YOU CAN'T MEASURE IT, YOU CAN'T MANAGE IT

The move from anecdote to antidote requires one key component: metrics. The title of this section pretty much says it all and contains more truth than most people are willing to admit. The reason that so much of what we do in relation to decision modeling is based on anecdotal evidence combined with experiential support is either because we don't understand the value of numbers or we don't trust the results. Think about how often we use in support of what we think, do, and say in our normal lives. If you have an appointment at 1:30 with a client at a particular location, you, like most of us, would go to MapQuest or use some other mapping tool to get a handle on the distance and time required to get to the appointment. Having experience with traffic flow at certain times, you would know how to convert the miles to the location into minutes (or hours). Knowing the ratio of miles to the gallon for the vehicle you are driving, you would be able to determine whether you needed to purchase fuel before you left.

If a new patient (as opposed to an established patient) is scheduled for a physician encounter, knowing that new patient visits take 20% longer than established patient visits, you might create a longer time slot for a new patient than for a follow-up visit. In fact, a detailed analysis of patient visit times by type of patient and chief complaint might well reveal a model for scheduling that would all but eliminate waiting time for both patients (time from check-in to exam room) and physicians (waiting for a patient to be in the room).

Imaging centers, like other businesses, make money based on volume of procedures performed. Knowing how long it takes to perform a procedure is critical in calculating the maximum number of procedures that can be performed in a given time period. Yet how often are measurements taken for turnaround time, a critical bottleneck for reaching maximum revenue? For example, if a procedure takes 30 minutes to perform (and we assume that it is pretty difficult to "rush" a procedure) and the center has eight working hours in which to operate, we might assume that the center could perform 16 of those procedures in a given day. This is not, however, the case, as there is time involved in getting the patients prepped, transporting them to the room, transporting them out of the room, and getting the room ready for the next procedure. If this entire process consumes 30 minutes, then the time for the procedure goes up to one hour and halves the number of procedures possible in the workday from 16 down to 8. Metrics allow us to "capture" the constraints in this process while analytics help us to get a better understanding on just what has occurred.

When we speak of data analyses, analytical modeling, statistical testing, and the like, for most folks, the hair will stand up on the back of their necks. This core response is usually due to their experiences in high school and college with the formulaic aspects of mathematics—the fearsome process of calculation. Fear not, however, because while important in its own right, that is not the focus of process improvement. Knowing how to measure a value, understand a statistic, and interpret work product is well within reach of every non-mathematician. But realize that without the ability to measure, the ability to manage and improve a process is unattainable.

THE THEORY OF CONSTRAINTS

The theory of constraints, while possibly not invented by Eliyahu Goldratt, was certainly made famous in his book of the same name.[4] The basic concept is simple: remove all constraints, and our ability to maximize efficiency approaches a limitless value. If you could remove all of the constraints involved in the patient visit cycle, you could theoretically see an infinite number of patients per day. Even within the most efficient of practices, however, time is a constraint that has a finite bottom limit; it takes some amount of time to see a patient, and there is a limit to the amount of time available in a day.

The goal, then, is to understand the idea of when a constraint is a bad thing and when it is a good thing. For example, having only one machine to perform complete blood counts in a busy practice is a bad constraint if it causes a back up of patients in the exam rooms reducing the turnover time and making physicians wait for a room. On the other hand, having the clinical staff rather than the physician review the intake form with the patient is a good constraint if it shortens the visit cycle for the physician, allowing him or her to see more patients for an increase in revenue.

A core concept in process improvement is the elimination of bottlenecks—the steps in a process that create a backup, adding to wasted time and resources and reducing customer (patient) satisfaction. A bottleneck is the result of a bad constraint; and, therefore, eliminating bad constraints results in a reduction of bottlenecks and a subsequent increase in efficiency and productivity. When a constraint is identified (usually through value stream mapping), the practice can determine if it is good or bad, required or redundant. For bad constraints, process improvement models call for the constraint to be promoted (elevated to a higher level to get it out of the way) or eliminated. The good news is, this usually opens a pathway for throughput, increasing overall efficiency and reducing cycle time. The bad news is, there is almost always another constraint waiting downstream.

References

1. Hammer M, Champy J. *Reengineering the Corporation: A Manifesto for Business Revolution.* HarperBusiness; New York, NY: 1994.
2. Hultman JA. *St. Anthony's Reengineering the Medical Practice: Profit Through Efficiency in a Medical Office Environment.* Reston, VA: St. Anthony Publishing; 1996.
3. Recklies O. Recklies Management Project GmbH. August 2001; www.themanager.org.
4. Goldratt EM. *Theory of Constraints: And How It Should Be Implemented.* Great Barrington, MA: North River Press; 1999.

THREE

Team Building

By Owen Dahl

CONTINUOUS PROCESS IMPROVEMENT as a concept cannot be implemented without the application of resources leading to the targeted outcome. These practice-based resources include time, talent, money, information, and materials. The most important aspect is the use of the right mix of individuals geared toward the improvement goal. These individuals will come together as a "high-performance" team that understands the goals, has the ability to take steps to accomplish the goals, and, finally, attains the successful outcome.

According to *Merriam-Webster*, a *team* is "a number of persons associated together in work or activity."[1] It is important to start with a clear definition of what a team is, and then move on to the components necessary to achieve the high-performance outcome that is desired. This chapter looks at the word "team," the administrative approach to structure of the team itself, the team process, and the "performance" aspects of the team.

A team might fit with the familiar phrase "Together everyone achieves more," which suggests that the whole is better than the sum of its parts. When we consider teams, we find that most of us work in teams to one extent or another. Teams work to solve more complex problems than one individual may be able to resolve. Teams are creative, they allow for access to many skills from the representatives, and, like it or not, they are always changing.

So why do we frequently work in teams? Teams allow the organization to understand the issues more thoroughly and become more creative in its approach through sharing of ideas, build stronger working relationships among the team members, allow team members to improve personally through learning new skills and enhancing existing ones, and become part of the solution. The organization will realize significant gains from each of these benefits when teams are utilized effectively.

TEAM DEFINED FURTHER

In looking to understand the idea of the team, Katzenbach and Smith identified five distinct types of teams.[2] As you consider these concepts, reflect back upon your own experiences, and see if you can identify with each of the types. Figure 1 identifies each of the team types as they relate to performance impact and effectiveness.

- **Working group.** This group comprises members who have come together for the purpose of sharing information, helping the individuals do their job better, and looking at best practices or perspectives that may help individuals accomplish their defined tasks. Here's a key to identifying a working group: there is no performance outcome from the group interaction. There is no real need for the members to interact to accomplish a team-based outcome. This may be confusing since *Merriam-Webster* defines a *group* as "a number of individuals assembled together or having some unifying relationship."[3] A working group can be a necessary and effective aspect of overall practice management. This could be the weekly meeting of the leadership when each individual informs others of what happened last week and what the current week looks like. The communication piece is necessary but is not performance oriented.

- **Pseudo team.** This is a group of individuals assembled to act as a team but who do not function is any way as a team. There is a performance objective, but there is no focus on it, and there is no interest in sharing a common set of goals. This is the weakest of all team types; in reality, the sum of its parts is less than the whole, and there is no contribution to

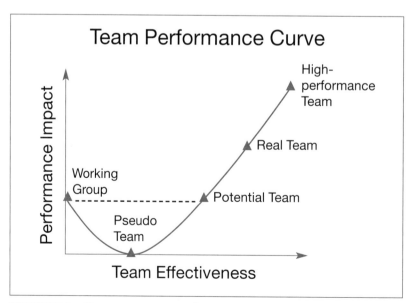

FIGURE 1. Team types on a performance curve.

the overall goals of the organization. This team searches for identity, has little or no leadership, and simply is meeting for the sake of meeting. In order to move to another level, there should be a clear focus on the performance objective and goals should be defined, roles assigned, and movement made toward accomplishment of the performance objective. This type of team is very costly in that there is a lot of expense with no measureable return for its efforts. The team must evolve into another type of team or be dissolved.

▪ **Potential team.** This team recognizes its performance objectives and is trying to improve. There is a need to clarify the goals and purpose of the team. Typically, there are many of these teams in organizations in which the individuals know things need improvement but can't quite get it together. This team may be similar in nature to a working group but has a definite performance objective. There is potential for organizational good through this type of team.

▪ **Real team.** The individuals in this type of team have and utilize complementary skills, are committed to the goal, and have an attitude of working together. This is clearly above the potential team level and is producing for the organization.

▪ **High-performance team.** These individuals have a deep commitment to one another and their personal growth as well as a clear understanding of and focus on the performance objective. The commitment transcends the team itself by outperforming its stated purpose. This type of team is the one that all teams strive to be. These teams have a clear understanding of their purpose, values, and relationships; know how to communicate; are flexible; receive recognition and appreciation from themselves and others; and have a high morale that can and will pervade throughout the organization.

To differentiate the common work group, which we see so often in practices, from teams, the key questions to ask are:

▪ Is there a performance objective or opportunity?
▪ Is there true interdependence upon each team member for the good of the team and for the individual?
▪ Is there share accountability—ownership of the team by its members?

Table 1 identifies key characteristics that will help the team define its type and lists the key steps necessary for the team to move toward high-performance team status. This should be discussed openly by the team members in one if not several of the team meetings.

TEAM ADMINISTRATIVE ISSUES

In establishing a team, the organization should receive an efficient and effective model for process improvement and problem resolution. The team that is properly functioning will

TABLE 1. Team-defining Characteristics[4]

Characteristic	Work Group	Real Team	High-performance Team
There is a significant, incremental performance need or opportunity.	If no, then it is a work group!	☆	☆
There is a joint commitment to a common mission.		☆	☆
There is a consensus on objectives.		☆	☆
There is an agreement on working approach.		☆	☆
There is true interdependency.		☆	☆
There is mutual accountability.		☆	☆
Members are committed to one another's personal growth and success.			☆
The team outperforms other similar teams and outperforms performance expectations.			☆

achieve those outcomes noted above in high-performance teams through increased morale, improved skills, better relationships, and improved problem-solving skills. And it will show others, especially management, that employees have great ideas and can effectively contribute to the success of the organization.

It is essential that ownership and management understand and accept the team idea as the most effective way to achieve improvement. They must support teams by providing an environment that allows "meetings" and understanding that improvements take time to become fully effective. If management expects solutions to improvement processes later the same day the problem is defined, a team process will not work. It is well known that individuals who are involved in developing the solution will commit to its implementation. Management must provide the resources necessary for the team to achieve. It must provide direction and support; clarify the problem and the performance objectives initially; provide an integrated plan that ensures consistency of overall organization objectives; and be available to reinforce these along the way. Positive recognition and reinforcement of the team process is essential to encourage its success.

Earlier we identified types of teams based upon an overview of team framework. In an organization that is seeking process improvement, there are specific team types that should be identified:

- Lean Six Sigma teams (see Chapter 2 for discussion on these terms) are formalized and trained with Lean Six Sigma leaders (e.g., Black Belts).
- Improvement teams are focused on specific areas or problems that are part of one department.
- Process improvement teams are usually multidisciplinary in nature.
- Project/taskforce/ad hoc teams are temporary in nature with one very specific objective identified.
- Self-directed teams are virtually independent of involvement from management but are given direction from management as to team objectives and thus are expected to meet specific goals in the desired time frame. The independent nature of these teams is such that members become leaders. These teams must have the confidence of management to continue to achieve their targeted outcomes.
- Cross-functional teams include representatives from different departments or areas in the organization. Members are chosen for the expertise and skill sets that they can bring to the project. Typically, these are major-problem-based projects for which significant resources are allocated by management. Some may refer to these as matrix teams with the idea of mixed levels of department or organization responsibility. These teams are key to successful organization-wide process improvement efforts.
- Quality teams provide a focus on improving quality within the organization, focusing on internal clinical areas for improvement projects. The organization focus on patient satisfaction, value-based processes, or successful patient outcomes are where these teams thrive.
- Natural work teams are departmental-based and address process improvement issues of that specific department. The department supervisor is typically the team leader. This is useful when there are specific departmental issues or to help the department develop improved working relationships.

All of these team types will seek to achieve either real-team or high-performance team status as they evolve through their specific functional outcome goals.

The first step in process improvement team project selection is to have an identified problem. As with most problem-solving processes, the true definition of the problem is often the most difficult task. Management may not have a clear definition of the problem, but it recognizes that there is a problem and accepts that a process improvement team is the most effective way to solve the problem.

Selection of team members may be done by management based upon recommendations from supervisors or others within the organization. This is often based upon the perceived scope of the problem, such as an organization-wide problem, a problem focused on patient quality, or a departmental problem, as noted in the discussion of the various specific types of teams. Someone must be identified as the process owner, which we will define shortly. Each member of the team will bring a specific set of skills, knowledge, and/or experience to the team; and as each individual buys into the goal or specific purpose of the team, he or she becomes a member.

Once the members are chosen, the first meeting is scheduled. It is important to have a well-defined agenda for this and subsequent meetings. The agenda should be distributed in advance to allow everyone to prepare based upon their area of expertise. Meetings should start and end on time. The role of the recorder should be assigned at the first meeting because documentation of the decisions, assignments, and outcomes is essential for ongoing communication to all interested parties and to keep the team focused.

We would suggest at the first meeting that the team develop a charter—a document that includes the following:

- Team members by name, department, and role (defined later);
- The specific purpose of the team—problem definition;
- The goals of the team;
- Structural issues such as when and where team meetings will occur;
- A commitment statement that all team members will agree to work toward the targeted outcome; and
- Identification of review dates to ensure that the process is monitored and that the project is on target.

Subsequent meetings then should be based upon an agenda that includes unresolved items, updates on assignments and status of activity, and new assignments should they be necessary. Recorded minutes of the meeting should be kept and provided to all members as well as other interested parties.

The size of the team is important to ensure efficient operation without duplication or excess use (waste) of resources. Teams should have no fewer than 3 members and no more than 15. For improvement teams, we recommend no more than 10 from a department; for quality teams, again no more than 10; cross-functional teams should include 8 to 12; and self-directed teams from 6 to 15.

Occasionally, the original team may not have been constituted correctly. The team may determine that is it lacking a certain skill set or knowledge level. However, it is important that this be a team-driven process and not something that is forced on the team—because the most efficient teams become dependent upon one another, and interference from management may be harmful. The team may also decide—due to poor attendance, lack of commitment to the project, personality conflicts, or violation of confidentially or other rules—that a member should be removed. This obviously is a tough situation; but keeping the long-term team goal in mind will make it easier to handle.

There are key roles for individuals that will constitute each team as follows:

- Champions are upper level managers that control resources and are specifically trained in process improvement techniques and strategies. They are supporters and not spies or detractors from the success of the team. They will be involved in the review process as the team evolves toward it targeted outcome.

- A facilitator is very important, but not a team member! The facilitator is from outside of the team, department, or organization. He or she should be trained in structure and process activities of a team.

- The team leader must provide direction and clarify assignments for all team members, act as a liaison to management, ensure that the administrative issues are dealt with appropriately and in a timely manner, enforce the charter, and work closely with (not against) all team members keeping a clear focus on the goals. The role encourages involvement and input. Occasionally, the designated team leader may give way to another for key activities of the process by recognizing specific contributions that the other member can make to the project outcome.

- A process owner is the expert on the process itself. He or she knows everything about the current process and can thus offer value stream mapping and other techniques or tools (which will be discussed in Chapter 5) necessary for successful outcomes. The individual may not be at the management level, but instead may be the organization billing expert for Medicare with the knowledge and the ability to communicate that knowledge effectively.

- Subject experts may have knowledge of the general area but not the intricate knowledge of the process owner. These may be other employees from the organization or department, or they could be brought in from outside the organization to provide needed information. This may be another biller or someone from a managed care company who is willing to help improve your internal processes. These individuals must be effective communicators.

- The recorder takes the minutes, copies them, and provides them to team members in a timely manner. The recorder also assists the team leader with the meeting agenda and circulation, and will follow-up with and encourage members to have their updates ready for the next meeting. A key role in the meeting itself is to keep time—when a topic is assigned a certain amount of time for discussion or it is time to adjourn, the recorder is the one who lets the leader know. The recorder may or may not be an official team member.

- No process improvement effort will be successful without the properly structured team with its purpose, members, and rules clearly understood. Teams working within these concepts will be effective, it they perform!

TEAM PERFORMANCE

Teams move through various stages as they evolve. These stages are defined here and offer the context within which any team type can achieve high-performance status. These stages were identified by Bruce Tuckman and are forming, storming, norming, performing, and adjourning.[5] For our purposes, we will focus on the first four stages with emphasis on the stage behaviors and feelings, and suggestions on how to deal with or improve that process.

Figure 2 suggests that there are key words to keep in mind as you review these stages. The knowledge that each team member brings as well as the accumulation of knowledge that occurs throughout the interaction and growth of the team must be always identified. The higher end of the scale suggests that the knowledge created through the process will lead to success. The other word that sticks out is the idea of trust. No team can grow without a basis of trust among the members.

Forming

In the initial stage, as you would expect, all members are introduced individually as well as to their expected role or contribution to the team. There is a discussion on the team charter and the expectations of the team. Members in their own way will transition from their individual role to one as a team member with its boundaries and expectations. They may test each member, especially the leader, either formally or informally. Discussions will typically be basic or superficial. There will be a lot of activity in the minds of members as they

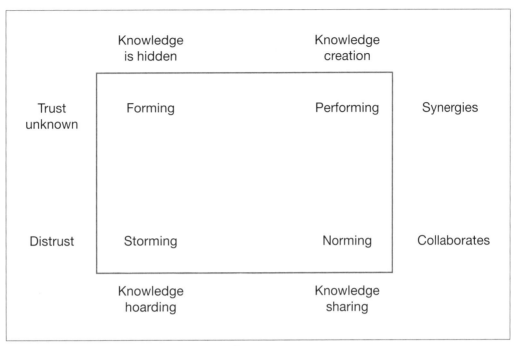

FIGURE 2. The stages of team process.[6]

attempt to assess what they are getting into. Typical behaviors evidenced in this stage will include lack of focus, difficulty in defining the problem at hand, varying levels of participation by members, resistance to the team-building process, and, often, ineffective decision making. Members will be excited, anticipating the process, as well as feel recognized for their selection as a team member. There may be suspicion, fear, and anxiety as well. Members will begin to feel part of the team but only partially so at this stage.

When teams are at this stage, it is important to identify roles that each member may play, either on a permanent or revolving basis. Meredith Belbin developed the context for these roles, which are categorized into three role areas:[7]

- **Action oriented:** Those who act here will typically help develop the ideas but more importantly can be counted upon to implement and complete the team project.
- **People oriented:** Those who act here are more "team players" who work with others in ways that will make the team more successful. They may also provide resources to achieve the goals
- **Problem-solving roles:** Those who act here are the thinkers and bring discipline and specific skills to the team, and assist in keeping the team on track based upon the initial objectives.

These roles will affect the culture of the team and should not be considered lightly. It is important for any team leader to recognize these roles and which individuals will occupy them.

Action-Oriented Roles

- **Shaper:** A shaper is a challenger, is dynamic, loves pressure, seeks to overcome obstacles, and is very committed to achievement of the desired outcomes. However, a shaper is subject to provocation and may offend others through his or her actions or comments. Occasionally, there may be more than one shaper, which could lead to significant conflict on the team.

- **Implementer:** An implementer is disciplined, reliable, and conservative. This member is practical and will work to achieve practical outcomes. He or she may be slower to accept new ideas and less flexible in dealing with changes.

- **Completer Finisher:** A completer finisher finds errors and omissions and conflicts in data, and is conscientious and anxious in his or her efforts to deliver assignments on time. This anxiety may cause the completer finisher to worry unnecessarily, and he or she may not be able to delegate well, which will lead to his or her desire to control the outcome.

People-Oriented Roles

- **Coordinator:** A coordinator is positive, mature, and confident; delegates well; excels at defining goals; and will promote decision making. This member may be seen by others as a manipulator and may be too good a delegator by passing off personal work. The coordinator may be quiet and reserved but also may be the team leader.

- **Team Worker:** A team worker is a cheerleader who supports team spirit, while being cooperative, mild mannered, a good listener, a builder, and averse to friction. Not a decisive person, a team worker will reserve opinions or comments to avoid offending another team member.

- **Resource Investigator:** A resource investigator is extroverted, enthusiastic, an opportunity seeker, articulate, excellent in negotiating, and friendly so as to create good contacts. Being overly optimistic may lead to lack of interest in the project once the initial phase is well underway.

Problem-Solving Roles

- **Plant:** A plant is very creative and imaginative; generates ideas; and is very good at problem solving, albeit a little unorthodox. A plant may not be a good communicator due to distractions and may miss things going on around the process or within the group.

- **Monitor Evaluator:** A monitor evaluator is logical and strategic, sees all options, is serious, has good judgment, and is objective. The monitor evaluator may not inspire others with an arrogant attitude and may be too critical of others by focusing too much on his- or herself.

- **Specialist:** A specialist displays single-minded dedication to the team, has lots of initiative, is knowledgeable, and brings good skills to the team. He or she will be narrow in focus and is highly technical in nature and approach.

Identifying these roles is critical for the ability for the team to move through all of the stages. It is important for the team to take the time necessary to become comfortable with each other. This may require more than one meeting and contact outside of the formal meetings themselves. It is important at this stage to establish all the ground rules and to keep focused on the purpose and goals of the team. Each team member should be trained on the processes and concepts of being a team member and be willing to participate. Members should encourage each other to share their thoughts and ideas. There are no bad ideas at this stage, there is little criticism, and the effort to "form" should be foremost in everyone's mind.

Storming

This stage brings out individual ideas, personal agendas, and different perspectives as to how to approach the tasks ahead. Arguments will surface! Members may be impatient and rely on their own experiences and knowledge rather than attempt to collaborate with the other members. Energy is wasted on issues rather than on making progress toward the targeted outcome.

Key behavioral issues evolve around the individuals and their effort to define their role and how the team will function. The arguments, hidden agendas, evolution of cliques, and poor decision making will be dominant. The exciting feelings from the forming stage will give way to resistance and focus on the individual.

Team problems that will surface here and may resurface at any stage include:

- **Floundering:** The team has unclear direction, and is overwhelmed with the nature and scope of the problem as well as delays in action. Here the team leader must maintain and reinforce the focus on the purpose and goals of the team effort.

- **Dominant Participants:** One or several individuals may attempt to take over or seek to make their point; they will interrupt and talk too much or too long. Structure and time limits will help, plus the enforcement of the rules noted in the charter will curtail these members.

- **Overbearing Participants.** Experts may attempt to take over and use their influence to control or steer the team in one direction (some of this may be legitimate). Team members should recognize this effort, and if not legitimate not tolerate this behavior. When legitimate, this is a time to allow for a new "leader" for this point to be well communicated and understood.

- **Negative Nellies.** These individuals defend their turf, are not able or willing to make contributions, respond to suggestions negatively, and make comments like, "We've already tried it, and it didn't work," or "That's a crazy idea." The team should work to refocus on alternatives that may work. It may also be important to determine if others are feeling the same way, and it is a team problem and not just one individual. Seek and channel new ideas to get the individual and/or team back on track.

- **Opinions as Facts:** Opinions and assumptions surface as facts, which leads to barriers to questioning the position taken. Members should be willing to challenge and ask for backup data—determine what is truly a fact. The team leader may have to take this member aside and seek clarification and help in restating the position.

- **Shy Members:** The quiet ones may support the team for a direction but may be passive/aggressive, so it is important to understand what is behind the shy action or approach. These nonparticipating members may not be a benefit to the team. Efforts should be made to involve these members, remove any threats, treat them with respect, and require them to take a position when the team votes on an issue. If they open up and participate, their contribution may be substantial. If they don't, then they may need to be removed.

- **Jumping to Conclusions:** The team may feel a need to reach a decision due to an agreed-upon deadline when in reality the process is still incomplete. Data may be missing. The time frame may be more important than the outcome. Take a serious look at the data; reconsider the time line based upon the level of discomfort or the focus on the date rather than the real solution. Review the priority and targeted outcome rather than make a decision that will not be in the best interest of the organization.

- **Attributions:** Inappropriate statements or positions are taken without other members of the team challenging what is being stated. These may be casual or psychological judgments. Here the team must challenge and seek clarification.

- **Put-downs:** Sarcasm—need more be said? One team member is commenting on or criticizing an individual or an idea. The team leader must take control and stop this behavior either in the team meeting or with the individual directly. The meeting focus should shift away from this topic to achieve refocus. It may be a great time for the facilitator to be contacted to address communication issues.

- **Wanderlust (drifting):** There is lack of focus, side conversations occur during the meeting, and there is difficulty keeping on task; everyone is seeing how big the issue is and chooses to be distracted. It is time to refocus, follow the agenda, and seek discussion points to get back on topic. This may be a very sensitive topic that no one wants to discuss; recognize that and shift, with the understanding that this topic will need to be discussed again in a different frame.

- **Feuding:** Negative comments such as, "I'm better than you," "I have given more suggestions than you," "Why you are on the team?" are made. Team workers and specialists may go along to relieve tension. The team leader must rise to the occasion and confront these individuals, usually best done in private! If the feud continues, the team member(s) may have to be replaced.

- **Risky Shift:** This is a willingness to take on unnecessary risks, going along with others, not fully understanding the resources available in the organization. The team should seek to understand the total picture including costs and any damage that may occur if a particular course of action is chosen; outside assistance may be necessary. A great question is, "If this were my money, how would I decide . . . ?"

The storming stage is a time to recognize that there will be conflicts! A conflict is:

"**a:** competitive or opposing action of incompatibles: antagonistic state or action (as of divergent ideas, interests, or persons); **b:** mental struggle resulting from incompatible or opposing needs, drives, wishes, or external or internal demands . . . the opposition of persons or forces that gives rise to the dramatic action in a drama or fiction."[8]

Storming may be a scary word or situation that could exist or surface in the organization or team process. This multifaceted look at the definition of the storming stage uses competition and opposition, then identifies individual perspectives, and ties it all together with dramatic action. It is very important to recognize that this can be both a difficult but also healthy situation for the team to deal with. A conflict may be preventable as well. A conflict may be based on an intellectual disagreement between team members. It may also be an emotional response to a statement, individual, or position taken. The team leader must recognize these scenarios and lead accordingly.

Conflicts are caused by:

- A misunderstanding;
- Differences in training or skills;
- Differences in values or morals;
- Differences in goals;

- Different priorities;
- Personalities; and
- Threats—direct or indirect—to the status, acceptance, individual.

At this point, it is important to emphasize that conflict is not necessarily negative. Positive things can result for the team during conflict through an increased understanding of the issues or of each other, a potentially stronger cohesive unit, and individual growth through an examination of how a person dealt with and responded to the conflict that surfaced. Thus a win-win situation can surface for the team and its individuals.

However, the negative side of conflict can be destructive to the team, its process, and sometimes its members. The sense of trust can be harmed, which then leads to a lack of cooperation among the members. Counterproductive behavior may result. It may be difficult if not impossible to forget the position or action of those involved, which may permanently harm the team outcomes. Forgiveness may be easier than forgetting, but the cloud lingers if the situation is not dealt with constructively.

There are many approaches to managing and resolving conflict. The approach identified here is based upon Thomas and Kilmann,[9] who have identified five main styles in dealing with conflict. Figure 3, which is based upon the Blake and Mouton managerial grid model, identifies the five styles on the X-Y axis of assertiveness and cooperation.

The five stages and their characteristics are:

- Competing-style members are those who take a firm stand and are committed to their desired outcome. They come from a position of power based upon position, expertise, or their ability to persuade others. This can be useful in an emergency or when a decision needs to be made quickly. It very often leaves team members who are unsatisfied, feel like losers, and may harbor resentment around the outcome.
- Collaborating-style members attempt to meet the needs of everyone who may be assertive but at the same time seek cooperation of all involved. This style works best when there is a need to bring everyone together to share their perspectives and when the situation is very important and the trade-off is not desirable.
- Compromising-style members try to at least partially satisfy all team members. All members, including the leader, are expected to give up something. This style works best when the conflict itself outweighs the targeted outcome, when there is a major deadline upcoming, and when all sides of the issue have equal strength.
- Accommodating-style members have a desire to meet the needs of others while sacrificing their own needs. This is clearly a nonassertive style that is useful when the issue is more important to the other side or when the current goal is peace rather than winning. It

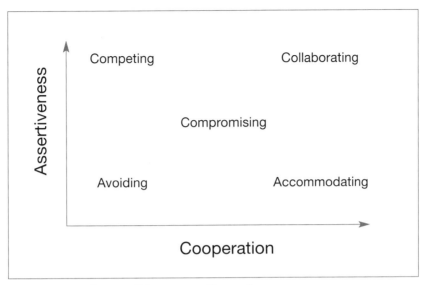

FIGURE 3. **Thomas-Kilmann conflict styles.**

may also be used to trade-off today's decision for an expected return tomorrow, however fragile that promise might be.

- Avoiding-style members have a desire to avoid conflict. These members delegate to others, accept another's decision, and don't want to hurt anyone's feelings. It can be a good style when a win is determined to be impossible, when someone has more knowledge, or when the issue is insignificant.

There is no one style that will work in every situation. Most individuals may identify with one style more than another. It is important to recognize that there are differences that may apply to specific situations.

In dealing with a conflict, the member or team leader should consider the basic problem-solving process (i.e., to identify a problem through a thoughtful assessment of the situation). Once information is gathered, then a style selection should occur that is deemed most appropriate. The next step, which is critical, is the need to negotiate to achieve what has been identified as the most viable solution for the resolution of the current situation, always keeping in mind the team's targeted outcome.

The storming stage is a great time to turn to the facilitator who may provide invaluable assistance in moving the team forward to the next stage. As noted previously, the facilitator is usually someone from outside the team who is trained in dealing with team processes and the accompanying dynamics. The facilitator should be able to provide an outside perspective on the issue at hand while assisting with keeping the team in focus. In addition, the facilitator should be able to assess the personalities and cultural issues involved and note who may need some skills or team building training. The facilitator will work closely with the leader throughout the stage. The facilitator should not be judgmental and should remain impartial to the situation at hand, not take sides or become the dominant player in the process. The open mind of the facilitator bringing objectivity to the team will go a long way in allowing the team to refocus and move forward.

One skill that all team members assume they have is the ability to communicate. It is the process that is necessary to build a solid team but it is also the one that can lead to conflict and loss of direction. Communication in its basic context requires a sender, a message, and a receiver. It can be written, verbal, or conveyed via body language in its chosen delivery method. The sender forms the message and chooses the delivery method. The receiver listens to what is being sent. To ensure that the message was received, a key that is often overlooked is the feedback from the receiver to the sender. Was the message clearly understood, resulting in further growth of the team process? Seeking ways to not only send but be assured that the communication process is complete will go a long way to team success. Communication is one of the most valuable tools for the process improvement team and should be a part of team development and training.

An organization is typically arranged in a vertical fashion that allows for downward and upward communication. The team leader will send messages to the team members that may include instructions, policies, assignments, and responsibilities. These messages will be sent to all members to ensure that there is consistency in actions that will follow. Upward communication acknowledges the message, provides feedback on the assignments and tasks undertaken, and provides everyone with a perspective as to where the team is now and where it is heading. This may best be done in writing because it may be necessary to not only inform the team leader but other team members, experts, and the facilitator.

The team may also have horizontal communication that flows between team members or others who may be involved in the process. Here it may be more beneficial for the clinical members to share information or the specialists to compare notes and not essential for everyone on the team. This is usually bi-directional in nature.

Communication is also formal and informal. The team leader or facilitator may need to communicate specific instructions, which is done in writing as a formal downward message. Formal communication may also be between members as data are shared that will assist the team toward its targeted outcome. Informal communication mostly occurs through a verbal exchange between members and can also be either downward or upward. The team charter and minutes represent formal communication. There are also organization-wide policies and procedures external to the team that must be understood and clearly followed.

As noted above in the storming stage, there will be conflicts. These very often can be eliminated or reduced if the members simply listen to the message that is being sent. We have two ears and one mouth, so a good rule of thumb is to listen twice as much as we talk! Listening requires practicing. Be patient with the sender and repeat back to the sender your understanding of the message, which will ensure that the communication process has been effective.

Helpful in the listening process is seeking understanding of the message and the story behind the message. A key technique is to ask why, not only once but up to five times. This drills down to the base of the message. The goal in understanding the message is to ask the right questions, not leading questions but probing through the "five why" approach. Don't hesitate to rephrase the message, and then pay close attention to the response to your response.

An important perspective to keep in mind is that when communication occurs, there is sharing. Speak slowly and clearly, choose the words that make the most sense to ensure the message is sent appropriately, avoid highly technical or multi-syllable words, and pause to allow the other member(s) to ask questions. Also, don't be afraid to ask for feedback or clarification of the message to ensure that it is clearly understood.

The storming stage can be the most difficult one to get through. It is also one that may surface again and again throughout the process. Therefore, the members, and especially the team leader, must be aware of the possibility of its rearing itself again and again. If there is adequate communication and constant attention on the purpose of the team, the number of reoccurrences will be reduced.

Norming

The norming stage occurs when the members reach a consensus, there is renewed enthusiasm for the task at hand, and the rough edges from the storming stage have been smoothed out. The members understand and accept the rules and the roles of each individual. Here the behaviors reveal improved attitudes, greater trust in each other, and a commitment to each other. There are actual accomplishments of the steps necessary to reach the targeted outcomes. There will be shared leadership as necessary, and individual and team growth occur. There is a level of comfort among members. Friendships are renewed or begun. There is a sense of cohesion around the purpose. The process improvement cycle really begins to see results through the attainment of key milestones that were targeted initially.

At this stage, decisions will be made as data continue to flow. It is necessary to define and accept structured ways to achieve consensus. Therefore, tools like brainstorming and voting, among others, will need to be discussed and selected.

It is also a time to be cautious. The good feelings may give way to "group think," which may not sound bad but could derail the focus and delay the process improvement cycle. There could be such loyalty as to cause a lack of openness in disagreeing with something that is happening. There could be more of a desire to keep the team together than to accomplish its results. The team itself could become the reason to exist rather than the stated goals of the team. In this scenario, the team may feel it is above criticism—that no one can contradict the process or current status; the team may fail to communicate as appropriate; a consensus could be reached too early; and the team itself, by its members, then must be protected from outside influence. If any of these symptoms occur, the team leader must stop and achieve a refocus among the team members.

More often than not, however, in the norming stage it is critical to share information and to make decisions. Brainstorming is a very effective method to generate a lot of good ideas that have come as a result of the data-gathering process that has occurred (see Chapter 4 for details). Steps included in the brainstorming effort include: define the issue; set a time frame; encourage anything and everything to come out and be recorded on a white board or flip chart; select a pre-determined number of ideas; determine criteria for evaluation; and set priorities on each item.

A mechanism that works well to reduce the number of items that are a result of a brainstorm process is to use a multi-vote procedure. Each member is given a certain number of votes (e.g., 10 items listed = 3 votes; 20 items listed = 5 votes; and 30 items listed = 8 votes each). If more items are on the list, determine votes accordingly. A second round of votes is taken based upon the outcome of the first; using the same idea of voting for more than one item until a desired number of items has been identified. Members can also "burn" their votes by using all votes for their favorite item rather than voting for several. A "weight" can be assigned based upon the number of "sticky dots" (tally points noted for each item, assign an ascending value, and calculate the number of votes to determine the winner[s]).

A variation on the brainstorming procedure is to use the nominal group technique developed by Delbecq and Van de Ven.[10] Here, an open-ended question is stated, and ideas about the question are written down, as opposed to openly stated as in brainstorming. After a set time period, time is called, and each member shares one idea at a time in a round-table fashion until all ideas are written on a whiteboard or flip chart without discussion. Then discussion occurs, and an anonymous vote is taken to select the best idea(s). This method allows for anonymity as well as allows for those who are quieter to have an equal say in developing the outcome. This process may appear to be too structured and may not allow for as much open discussion.

The norming stage, then, shows significant progress based upon analysis of data, open sharing, and a reasonable decision making/selection process. There should also be an evaluation of the team process with open discussion. It would be beneficial to recognize small wins to the group, and interim reports may be submitted to management. There may also be relationships built with others outside the team based upon their involvement with the data gathering or expertise that is offered to the team.

Performing

Stage four is where things really happen; a real or high-performance team emerges. Members work through their personal issues and those with others, the group process is clearly understood and managed well by all, and there is significant creativity where the concept of the whole is greater than the sum of its parts occurs. Closer personal relationships based upon trust and respect are also formed. There are feelings of self-acceptance, appreciation of strengths, and acknowledgement of weaknesses, and clarity and direction result.

In this stage, a work product with a plan and recommendations for direction as well as implementation emerges. The outcome will need to be formally written as well as developed in such a way to give a presentation to management and or others in the organization. The outline of the document and presentation should include:

- Present the problem statement.
- List the purpose and goals determined initially.
- Identify the time line and key milestones that occurred along the way.
- List the process that occurred including the steps used to gather data, the analytical process, and other administrative items that proved beneficial and necessary.
- Note the benefits, risks, opportunities, and resources required.
- Present an action plan for implementation of the recommendations that have been noted.
- Use charts, graphs, and appropriate visual aids necessary to ensure that all who are receiving the information gain a clear understanding of the recommendations and implementation plan.

It is important to recognize that these stages are labeled one through four and have been presented here sequentially. This is not always how the team will evolve. There may be times when new members are added or others removed, meaning that the team has reverted back to the forming stage. There can always be conflicts or behavior role changes that will cause delays or lead to other issues. The norming or performing may not be as smooth as originally projected. Therefore, the team members, and especially the team leader and/or facilitator, must constantly be assessing the team process to ensure that it is maintaining its focus and that the bumps in the road are small and cam be smoothed out or eliminated.

The team may be asked to stay together to carry forward with the implementation so full adjournment may not be a direct outcome.

Adjourning

Tuckman added a fifth stage, that of adjournment. This stage may or may not be a result of any of the team models discussed. If adjournment or dissolution of the team does occur, it is recommended that there be one final meeting to review the entire process. These points should be memorialized and shared with the facilitator and management. Lessons learned from each team when shared throughout the organization will lead to improved team processes in the future.

It is essential for a successful process improvement effort to utilize the human resources available internally and externally to the organization leading to the successful achievement of the targeted outcomes.

References

1. Merriam-Webster's Online Dictionary; www.merriam-webster.com/dictionary/team.
2. Katzenbach JR, Smith DK. *The Wisdom of Teams*. Boston, MA: Harvard Business School Press; 1993.
3. Merriam-Webster's Online Dictionary; www.merriam-webster.com/dictionary/group.
4. Kane M. Distinguishing Teams from Work Groups Is Critical. LeaderValues; www.leader-values.com/content/detail.asp?contentDetailID=76.
5. Tuckman BW. Developmental sequence in small groups. *Psychological Bulletin.* 1965;63:384-399.
6. Clark D. Matrix Teams. The Performance Juxtaposition Site; www.nwlink.com/~Donclark/leader/leadtem2.html.
7. Belbin Team-Role Summary Sheet. Belbin.com; www.belbin.com/content/page/1950/Belbin_Team_Role_Descriptions.pdf.
8. Merriam-Webster's Online Dictionary; www.merriam-webster.com/dictionary/conflict.
9. http://kilmann.com/conflict.html
10. Sample JA. Nominal group technique: an alternative to brainstorming. *Journal of Extension.* 1984; www.joe.org/joe/1984march/iw2.html.

FOUR

Project Management

By Owen Dahl

A KEY PART OF ANY PROCESS IMPROVEMENT effort is understanding that processes go on forever but the effort to fix them or to expand them involves a short-term look at the bottlenecks or new opportunities. This is where the concept of project management comes into play.

Let's start with a review and expansion of key terms. Previously, we defined a *process* as a series of steps and actions that are taken in order to accomplish something. Basically this is everything that we do both personally and in the management of the practice. Washing your hair in the shower is a process from turning on the water to applying the shampoo to rinsing and drying. Each step along the way is part of the process designed to accomplish the goal of clean hair. One of the major purposes of this book is to provide tools for the application of process improvement: can you wash your hair differently to achieve a better outcome?

As we consider the improvement idea, how do we identify and select the step or steps that are bottlenecks or that need to be improved to provide a better outcome? This is where the idea of project management enters the equation. The Project Management Institute identifies the process of project management as shown in Figure 1. The model indicates that the key component is the plan. There is a need to develop components of the plan and to return to each component after inclusion in the plan for monitoring and control with regard to each component's contribution to the project as a whole.

A project is simple compared with a process. A project is a finite effort to fix a problem or to create a new service, while a process is a continuous set of steps necessary to achieve the goal. A successful project effort will result in an improved process or the implementation of the service desired. In order to deal with a project, there is a need for project management, which is a process! Confusing? A successfully managed project includes planning, organizing, and managing all aspects—resources, tools, deploy-

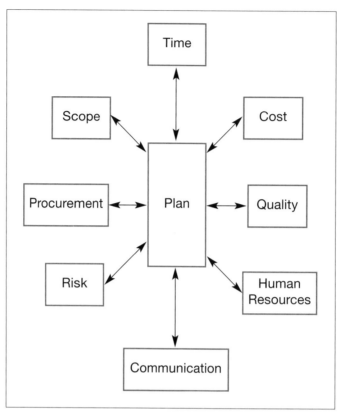

FIGURE 1. Project Management Institute project plan model.

ment platforms, etc.—to accomplish the targeted outcome. The key here is to ensure that the right resources—time, staff, and budget—are allocated to the project effort in an optimal way to achieve the goal.

There are many definitions of project management, but this one fits well with the concept that we discuss here: "Approach to management of work within the constraints of time, cost, and performance requirements."[1] As mentioned in Chapter 2, removing constraints coupled with the ability to maximize efficiency will produce exceptional results. The goal of project management then is to address constraints of time, cost, and performance to achieve those results.

So project management is a process that helps the team organize and focus to:

- Select the right project at the right time;
- Stay focused;
- Create specific solutions to the identified specific problem; and
- Determine if and when success is achieved.

In many practices, the approach to a problem that surfaces is to quickly jump to the solution without fully understanding the problem. Occasionally this actually results in a positive outcome, but more often than not what really happens is that another problem is created. Let's assume that the major "process" in any clinic is the patient visit, which can be divided into five basic steps (see Figure 2). The patient checks in and waits. Then at some point (stated this way to challenge you to think about the wait time issue seen in most clinic experiences), he or she is brought to the medical area by the medical assistant (MA). The MA interviews the patient, checks the patient's weight and vital signs, and escorts to the patient to the exam room. Again there typically is a wait time, some of which may be unacceptable to the patient. The physician or mid-level provider sees the patient, the real reason for the visit. After this step of the process, the patient returns to the MA's attention either in the exam room or in another area. Post-physician activity results in a prescription, test or appointment scheduling, or further instructions for care and treatment. Finally, the patient leaves the clinical area and returns to the front desk for discharge.

At any of these steps, there can be a "defect" or a "lag." A *defect* means that something is wrong, broken, or missing, such as the requested test results are not on the patient's chart and there is a need to scramble to find the information so the physician may complete the patients visit, or the proper needle is not in the exam room for a patient receiving an injection. The *lag* is the time delay that may occur during any of these steps.

Caring for the patient in an efficient and timely manner results in a positive experience and an increased likelihood of compliance with the treatment plan and a return to the practice should the need arise again in the future. The patient then becomes the key stakeholder in our process, a point that we must keep in mind with any and all project management efforts (Figure 2).

Projects succeed when there is real buy-in from the project champion, team leader, executive management, and the process owner that there is a need to fix or add something to the practice to better meet the needs of the patient stakeholder. This recognition is translated into a clear understanding of what needs to be done and the resources required to accomplish the goal. Effective planning and a realistic, as opposed to idealistic, approach are essential as well.

Is your practice ready for project management? This is a question not to be taken lightly! The starting point is the mission or vision of the practice. Is there consensus as to the purpose and a clear understanding among all owners as to why the practice exists? Without this, it will be impossible to ensure that resources are allocated toward fixing an issue. Anyone can perform quick fixes without any real targeted long-term outcome, but does

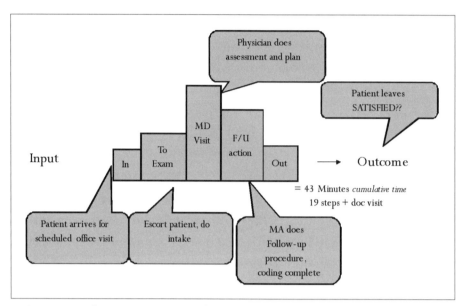

FIGURE 2. **Clinic visit process. F/U, follow-up; MA, medical assistant; un, unknown**

this really contribute to the success of the mission? Is there a willingness on the part of everyone to actually implement a true project management program?

Next is a critical look at the practice. What does it do well? Where are the problems or bottlenecks? Is the practice efficient or could it become more efficient? Are there resources available and are you willing to commit those resources to solve process issues? Does the practice have the capacity to actually make the change—balance the mission with the resources to grow and improve? Can you identify constraints that may affect the outcome of any project and can these constraints be removed?

If you addressed each of these questions and have determined that there is a positive perspective for implementation of project management to achieve continuous process improvement in the practice, then you should:

- Recognize the importance of the customer;
- Realize that speed, quality, and cost are universally linked;
- Believe that variation must be minimized;
- Know that bottlenecks need to be identified and removed;
- Use data and metrics as a key to decision making;
- Understand the importance of teams;
- Recognize that every employee, in one way or another, needs to be engaged in the process improvement strategy; and

▪ Turn to outside assistance when necessary to keep from stagnating.

Project management is not something that just happens. It is not the situation that one day the practice leaders decide, "We will now use project management as our preferred way to proceed into the future." It really requires a change in culture. This requires a plan, a lot of discussion on the issue(s) facing the practice, and a desire to change and to move forward into the future. It is not something that you can look at and say, "We will get a substantial return just by changing our philosophy." One of the significant benefits is the framework that is developed; this process can be replicated. This will result in savings of both time and money. These processes will not have to be reinvented each time a new problem surfaces. Communication to all or key team members is facilitated and enhanced by all understanding the process. It requires a clear understanding on the part of the practice leaders and a resulting commitment to the concepts that are being addressed throughout this book.

PROJECT MANAGEMENT LIFE CYCLE

A project has what is often referred to as a "life cycle," which is depicted in Figure 3. The first step is the identification of a problem. Once identified, the cycle goes through the clarification step, which we have identified as the project charter. Then the work begins. And once the milestones are accomplished and the project goal is achieved, the project is closed.

The team leader and the team members have different areas of emphasis in the entire life cycle. The team leader meets with the champion and anyone who may have an influence

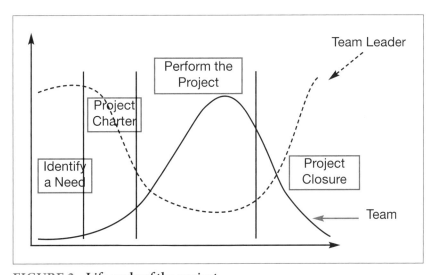

FIGURE 3. Life cycle of the project.

on the direction and outcome of the project. The planning phase is critical. It will identify the need for the project and define the details noted in the project charter. The charter is a key tool in the overall plan—designed to keep everyone in focus. Once the plan is in place, the workload shifts to the team members to accomplish the tasks and meet the milestones. The team leader becomes more of a coordinator, ensuring that the work is being done adequately and in a timely manner.

Identify a Need

The first step in the life cycle of a project—identify a need—is the most difficult. How do you do it and make sure that it is an appropriate project to which to devote practice resources? For example, you could pick an easy one—it may be "blatantly obvious" that you constantly have complaints about wait time. The practice could decide that this problem needs to be reviewed through the project concept and with a project team. Another option is to consider problems or expansion goals through a brainstorming process. Perhaps the practice leadership team regularly meets and decides that one of the meetings or part of each meeting will be used to do a review of the processes currently done in the office. The team then goes through a formal brainstorming process (more fully described in Chapter 5). The other major source of issues would come from your practice management or electronic medical records system potentially through your practice dashboard or other reports. Perhaps you have identified a major issue with denials from one of your major payers. This then looks like a project that needs to be addressed.

Recalling the definition of project management, it is important in identifying the need to remember the constraints that are associated. It may be that Dr. A will not change. Or perhaps Dr. B has always done things that way, and there will be several constraints associated with addressing this/his particular problem. The key in project selection is to remember the mission of the practice and to understand the impact of the current situation and the risks/rewards associated with the effort to solve the problem identified.

Remember that any project selected will take time and require resources. Therefore, it will be important to select a project that warrants attention. Parameters that are necessary to consider when reviewing selected projects should:

- Meet the goals of the majority of the stakeholders;
- Have a broad appeal to the practice;
- Be relatively simple to manage;
- Show some initial benefits as a way to ensure buy in and excitement;
- Be able to be controlled by the team;

- Meet financial and resource constraints; and
- Have definable and attainable start and finish dates.

Problem/Project Definition

We now find ourselves in the problem definition phase of the life cycle. A problem statement like "patients wait too long" is not sufficient. It is very important at this point to take time to clearly define the problem. It may be that new patients are complaining that the paperwork requirement is too lengthy and difficult to follow. This is a more clearly stated problem. Therefore it is easier to identify team members, time frame, and resources to address the problem than the more general the statement of patients wait too long.

In this definition phase, there may be a gap identifying where the practice currently is and where it would like to be. This gap indicates that there is a problem and that there will be significant effort required to meet the overall problem solution. This can be defined and developed without specific metrics as this point. However, the goal of identifying the specific metrics will follow.

What gets measured gets done; you've no doubt heard this before! If the current measure is that 65% of the new patients have complained that it takes too long on the first visit, obviously that is an unacceptable number. The goal could be that no one complains or a continuous improvement goal of 50% of patients complain, then 25%, then 10%, with the milestones achieved as measureable points.

It is then possible to measure the patient satisfaction and/or financial return from this effort. Patients are seen on a more timely basis, and more new patients are seen, which means more time for other things and/or increased income. These are outcomes that clearly will excite everyone involved in the practice!

As we look at the problem statement, each time one is created compare it to this checklist:

- Does it stipulate who, what, when, and where?
- Does it avoid the cause of the problem and identify the issue only?
- Does it stipulate the difference between here and there?
- Does it use quantifiable measures?
- Is it declarative and not stated as a question?
- Does it address the problem or the "where it hurts" aspect of the practice?
- Does it address the cause rather than the symptoms?

In considering what a physician does every time a patient is seen, we can see a major effort to clearly define a problem through the process of asking questions, seeking lab or other diagnostic feedback, documenting the findings to help clarify the picture, and then outlining the available alternatives to use to treat the patient. If the physician jumps to treat a symptom before taking time to truly identify the problem, there may be an unacceptable outcome and a total risk of failure. This same process must be applied to this phase of the life cycle—define and understand the problem.

Project Charter

The next step in the project life cycle is the project charter, which is a key portion of the planning phase. In this case, a form (document) is recommended as a guide that will enable effective communication of the many components of the charter. (See Figure 4 for a model.) According to Morris, "Charters can take many forms, but at a minimum it should contain a scope statement and target dates and cost, and establish the authority of the project manager. Without this document, it could be very difficult to get any decision made or run a successful project." [2] So why do you need a project charter? It provides a structure! The structure is not just for one project but for every project that is implemented in the practice. The use of the form develops the plan, further defines the goals, and records the targeted milestones and tasks as assigned. Once the format is used, it will more easily be identified as a tool to assist in the project management process.

Initially the charter is developed by the team leader, champion, and key executive(s) of the organization. This initial effort is to review the project purpose or scope and to identify the desired goal with the deliverable(s) necessary to attain that goal. Remember one of the keys is to recognize the key stakeholder(s) and their goals/needs. Discussion will include potential team members, the resources, and the time frame necessary to achieve the goal.

Fill in the fields of the charter with the following ideas:

- The project name should identify the main aspect or idea of the project. The start date should be clearly identified.
- Team members should be listed. This was covered in the previous chapter, so please refer to it for more details on who assumes the appropriate roles. To review however, the keys are the team leader, facilitator, and stakeholders. Once these are identified, it will be easier to communicate to, from, and with top management or the physician owners to complete the charter itself.
- The problem statement is listed as defined by the project champion and process owner. Team members may also be involved in the development of this statement. At the very least, everyone must clearly understand the project definition, sometimes referred to as the project scope.

Project Name		Start Date
Team:	Leader	
	Members	
	Facilitator if needed:	
	Stakeholders	
Problem statement or business case		
Purpose/goal (business need)		
Objectives (measurable)		
Assumptions		
Risks		
Deliverables		
Boundaries		
Task	Assignment/duties	Due Date
Milestones		
Communication strategy		
Budget		
Final presentation	Who:	Date
Recommendation		
Accepted/revision:		Date:

FIGURE 4. Project charter.

- The purpose or overriding goal must be clearly stated. This also clearly defines the scope of the project.

- The objectives may also be added. It is possible to have the goals and objectives in the same field depending upon how broad or segmented the problem definition is. In either case, the goals and objectives must be measureable with a metric that is understood and attainable. The baseline measure may be included in the problem definition or in the purpose statement. It should not be included with the listed objectives.

- Assumptions should be addressed. These might include items such as time limitations on meetings, lack of resources available, and that there will be non-team members involved in providing advice to the project.

- A project risk identifies those items that may cause the project to fail or what might create issues that would affect the outcome. These may include documents, policies and procedures, and new steps in a process.

- Deliverables are expected outcomes, tangible or intangible, as part of the project.

- A boundary is created to ensure that the focus of the project is maintained and that interference and input from outside these parameters may have a negative impact on the project as defined. This also defines the dates for the beginning and the end of the project itself. Boundaries should also further clarify the whos, roles, and expectations/ parameters of the team members. One of the key tools to assist here is SIPOC (Suppliers, Inputs, Process steps, Outputs, and Customers; see chapter 5 for more discussion on the SIPOC diagram). SIPOC helps to create the "picture" and further define the boundaries as to who is involved and what is expected. Remember that there may be some real constraints such as finances, availability of resources, etc. that will create boundaries that must be accepted.

- Tasks are developed and assigned to the team members, and due dates noted as part of the overall planning process. A task can be considered a subset of activities that are part of the project itself. In most cases, tasks don't stand on their own, and each task that is deemed necessary relates to another task in the project. Therefore, when we look at the task list noted on the project charter, the key tasks may be identified, while several others would be identified in the project management tools, which are discussed in the section on project charters later in this chapter.

- A project milestone is not a deliverable but rather a checkpoint in the process showing the progress made. Usually a point in time is set when a report is given on the status of the project—a report on the progress to achieve the outcome. Specific dates that are identified to assist in the accountability of the process should be identified in this section of the charter.

- The project charter details the strategy of who, when, and what will be communicated. Remember that one of the most important aspects of any process is the communication component. The team should communicate with the project champion on a scheduled basis. It is also important to recognize the need to communicate with the team members. Minutes taken and distributed as well as updates through verbal or e-mail to all other team members on the status of the milestones and/or deliverables as assigned will be key to the success of the project.
- The financial consideration through a budget can be as detailed as defined by the organization. This means that the man-hours assigned and expended can be tracked or that the budget can identify any outside assistance, copying costs, costs for securing additional information, or anything of this nature that should be considered in the budget component. The budget is a guide and offers another opportunity for the practice to assess the overall effectiveness of the project charter as a tool.
- The final presentation to the project champion culminates the entire project. This should be in a format defined by the practice. It could be a formal PowerPoint presentation or a simple written summary and set of recommendations. In any event, it should include the final set of recommendations by the team as defined and agreed to in the problem definition.
- The recommendation section is actually two parts.
  — Part 1 is a summary of the findings and the actual recommendations related to the improvement or implementation of the changes or new product/service being offered as a result of the project.
  — Part 2 is a detailed summary of what went right, what could be improved, and an honest assessment of the use of the project charter form and process.
- Acceptance/revision is a place for signature of the project champion. This represents the completion of the project per the project charter. If accepted, fine. If the outcome as presented is *not* acceptable to the champion, it may/will be necessary to develop another charter.

Another key aspect of the project charter is the issue of determining priority and the allocation of resources. One example of a project charter being implemented in a large practice included such things as everyone on the management team accepting the recommendation and use of the tool. This evolved to several key managers being assigned to teams. Individuals were either team leaders or team members on too many teams, and the entire system bogged down. Some management team members really liked and accepted the idea while others did not. The practice administrator had significant problems in tracking all of the project charters placed on her desk.

Therefore it became important to develop a system of monitoring and determining priorities of any and all projects. Back to the first line of the charter, the project title was essential to define and clearly represent the intent of the project. The practice intranet contained a folder that identified all project charters alphabetically. In this way, anyone who had access to the folder could review and understand the status of any project, in particular his or her own projects. It became a self-policing approach. In addition, the practice administrator was able to review the status and if necessary adjust the priority and resources applicable to the projects. This could be done without meetings because the details of the project status were communicated to all based upon the communication strategy. Once the initial details were worked out, the entire system became a smooth, effective process to control the projects designed to improve the processes!

Before leaving the charter, there are areas that warrant additional discussion.

Goals/Objectives

The project must have a well-defined purpose or goal. A project can be used for new items to be added to the practice such as an ultrasound system or implementing ePrescribe. In both cases, the overall goal would be successful implementation with a revenue stream expected. A fix project might be to reduce the overall time a patient spends in the office from 62 minutes to 45.

The objectives to accomplish the goal of a new revenue stream would include the development of a financial pro forma, an installation plan, a training plan, and a method to monitor effectiveness. The objectives for the patient flow process might include to identify the key bottlenecks, determine the most effective fix, implement, and follow-up. The first objective might be to reduce the total time from 62 to 55 minutes in a 90-day window. A continuous improvement approach would follow with another review following the 90-days, and the cycle would start over again.

Another common term used when talking about goals and objectives is *deliverable*. A deliverable can be the end result or product that is produced by the project.

Resources and Cost

"This idea is great, except we don't have time to designate staff to work on projects, they barely have enough time to do what their job descriptions require now. There is too much pressure on us to produce to try to deal with involvement with a project!" This has been said or thought more often that anyone can count.

We must go back to the point of the mission statement and the fact that the practice exists to meet the needs of patients who seek care. Can the practice survive in the long run without developing a philosophy of change and continuous improvement? This is why it is important to identify and assign the right staff to the project. The right staff means the skill that an individual brings, the available time, and the ability to relate to others on the team (see the storming stage in previous chapter). The right number of staffers is also critical, with too few meaning that the goal time may not be met, too many may lead to inefficiencies in the process!

Direct staff time may not be the only resource. It is possible when doing a project that there will be disruption of the normal process. In a wait-time study, does the support staff have to stop and note the time at each stop along the process either manually or as part of the electronic medical record? If so, there should be consideration given to a disruption factor.

In some cases, it may be necessary to train team members. This could involve training on project management or orientation to the concept. It would be wise to have a well-defined orientation program for anyone who is new to project management and who is expected to participate in the process. There may also be a need to train the staff on the tools that will be utilized. One team member may have a very specific task to accomplish, and additional training will be necessary to bring the individual to the level of competence desired. All these are costs that must be considered.

A project management example program could very easily be the development of the tools, definition of terms, and the presentation materials necessary to orient new team members to the project management idea. This could actually be the first project for the practice!

It is entirely possible that the project may require resources in the form of tools, software, utilization of a facilitator, supplies, or other items. These must be considered as the project is defined. There will be a cost associated with these resource requirements as well.

It is important to develop a realistic budget for the project. How much staff time at what hourly cost will be needed? Then add in the cost of the other necessary resources. In consideration of this, it may actually be too costly to begin a project! The return on investment may actually reveal that the cost to fix the problem is greater than the cost to continue as is; this is highly unlikely, but possible.

Here's a key word that must be put in context: procurement. When you think of procurement, you think of buying something such as a new ultrasound machine. You are going through a process and making a decision that something needs to be purchased. This also applies to routine items like office or clinical supplies. Therefore, the idea of procurement must be considered when developing the budget to ensure that the timing of the purchase, the bidding process, the delivery, etc. are consistent with the project time lines.

Another key to procurement is human resources. It may be that as team leader you have a particular individual in mind to assist with the project. It may be necessary to "negotiate" with that individual's direct report to secure release from normal duties to assist as a team member on the project. This may be easier said than done. Respect for the project since it is part of the overall culture of the practice is what one individual has to think about. While on the other hand, it will be necessary to consider the time required to complete the project and the total time away from regular duties for the employee. This balancing act and the overall time demands contribute significantly to the risk associated with the completion of the project.

Risks

Risk, when simply defined, suggests that the project or components of the project may be exposed to uncertainty. This uncertainty is what risk management is all about. Every project undertaken is a risk in that it might fail; this is an internal risk because it relates to the project itself. An external risk is one that is outside of and may result from the project. If we assume (here we have the idea of making and clearly understanding the assumption section of the charter) that the new ultrasound machine will be safe and effective we may be missing something. What happens if the system has a malfunction and causes an injury to the patient? Patient safety is not necessarily directly related to the project decision but the risk of outcomes might cause more issues without the practice having thought this through in the project process itself.

Anytime that a date is specified in the project plan, there is a risk that the date may not be met. It is therefore important to understand all aspects that may have a direct impact on the project—internal risk. The team leader addresses the risk potential in the plan and remains acutely aware of it throughout the process. The right staff members, their experience (or lack thereof), software, communications, and lack of supplies or equipment present a risk to the successful completion of the project.

The team leader should follow a simple process:

- Analyze each risk related to the project;

- Monitor and adjust those risk scenarios that surface that can be effectively managed; and
- Prioritize and remove all low-end risks that can be easily eliminated or repaired.

Awareness of the potential for a risk is critical. It is possible to mitigate or to deal with a risk before it actually becomes one. This involves planning and the ability to identify the potential of the risk occurring.

Monitoring a risk requires a system based upon awareness and then the ability to track what may be or is occurring. A long-term project will have more potential for risk than a short-term one, and therefore requires more attention to be paid to the risk itself. As you monitor a project, you may find that the risk is not as great as once thought and therefore does not require intervention. A simple question as to the tolerance for the variance of the risk occurring and its outcome may allow for the project to proceed without any intervention. As monitoring progresses, it may be discovered that the initial time frame was not calculated properly, there may be other tasks that take priority over another one, the wrong person may have been assigned to the task, or there may be technical glitches. Any one of these at anytime will have an effect on the outcome of the project.

A graphic may help complete the picture on the idea of risk management (see Figure 5). The approach to managing any real or perceived risk is the same that you find in problem

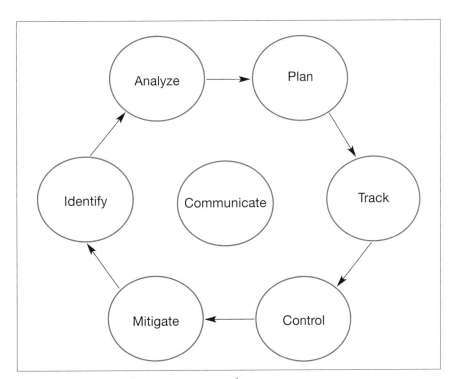

FIGURE 5. **The risk management cycle.**

solving. Be aware that the keys are either to control or mitigate it and to make sure that everyone involved is communicated with adequately. The cycle issues are:

- **Identify.** Search for and locate risks before they become problems.
- **Analyze.** Transform risk data into decision-making information and metrics.
- **Plan.** Transform decision-making information into decisive action.
- **Track.** Monitor risk indicators and actions continuously.
- **Control.** Adjust for deviations or variances from what was planned.
- **Mitigate.** Reduce the potential impact of the risky situation.
- **Communicate.** Provide feedback to all involved.

The team leader should establish a system of prioritizing risks by using a number or alpha designation. A high risk, designated H or 1, would indicate a substantial probability of the risk having a major impact on the project. A medium risk, designated as M or 2, might indicate a lower risk but still something that must be monitored. A low risk, designated as L or 3, might prove to be inconsequential and therefore requires no intervention. Using a designation system will help with awareness and the ability to pay close attention if required.

Beyond the issue of risk, experience has shown that there are typical problems associated with project management:

- Too many people are involved with decision making and want things done their way and/or in their time frame. It is possible to have too many leaders, either formal or informal in nature, that will have an impact on the project outcome.
- There is a problem in timing the beginning or the targeted end of the project. The recent economic downturn may have forced a delay in new project implementation. There may be a significant cash flow issue or layoff by a major employer and its self-funded health plan. These issues would impact a project dealing with what had been increased patient flow.
- There is a change in team members. These changes can be quite problematic, especially when members either resign or get pulled away due to time demands of the project interfering with what is perceived as a more important task.
- The project is delayed due to priority issues with other aspects of the practice. The project was perceived to be a very high priority, but all of a sudden staff is pulled, resources are taken away, or something happens to delay it for a period of time.
- The project receives too high a priority. This is the opposite of delay, and the expectation is that it will be done tomorrow. The scope of the project along with the plan is not well thought out, and the entire project is doomed to failure.

- The team issues noted in the previous chapter surface. Team members don't get along or there are one or two who subvert the entire project due to their own agenda.
- A repeat project is undertaken since the first time there was a failure. There may be less desire to be involved or to put the necessary effort into achieving the goal. The project may be doomed to fail. Or it is possible to have identified enough issues in the revised plan that the project could be very successful. The momentum to try again will have an impact on the outcome.
- Group think may take over. Everyone either gets along so well *or* they almost become one and lose their objectivity, and the project ends up in a different direction than what it should have been.

The practice should consider contingency plans that include the needs, resources, techniques, responsibilities, and requirements to complete the project. Then an identification of the needs associated with the risks such as systems, alternative plans, and analytics may have a way of reducing the risk. The practice may also develop contingency plans in the analysis phase based upon simulations, decision analysis, and performance tracking.

The overriding component of risk management is how to handle the risk. Any risk situation can be avoided, controlled, accepted, transferred, or mitigated depending upon the interpretation of the project champion or team leader, or input from team members. Any of the risk-handling techniques will work and should always be kept in the forefront of any project management thought.

Milestones

We have not addressed boundaries to any great extent; however, these are important in terms of risk issues. These are really checkpoints represented by specific dates with the idea to stop and review the status of the project and to determine if any schedule or resource changes are necessary to accomplish the targeted results.

Communication

How does the stakeholder know that the project has achieved its first milestone? Or better yet, how does the project champion approve the project charter with its required resources, defined budget, and the time frame necessary to achieve the project goals? This is accomplished by a well-thought-out effort to communicate. Regularly scheduled meetings with appropriate attendees are a necessary component. The use of e-mail is another. Recording minutes of each team meeting with circulation of the minutes to the right staff is essential.

The key point is that it is necessary to include communication guidelines in any plan, and they must be followed. Very often projects either fail or don't achieve their optimum outcome because there was poor communication to the right people at the right time.

Schedule

The project charter having now been introduced, it must include and be supported by a truly functional plan. The scope of the project is outlined with the project goals and objectives. One of the key sections of the charter or of any project effort even without a charter is the assignment of responsibilities and the allocation of resources. If there is not adequate time spent on planning, the odds of success for the entire project diminish.

There are several tools that are available that start with the Work Breakdown Structure (WBS) and move to and through options such as Program Evaluation and Review Technique, Critical Path Method flow charts, or Gantt Charts. We will address each in this section.

WBS is a tool developed to assist in the planning phase of project management. This "structure defines tasks that can be completed independently of other tasks, facilitating resource allocation, assignment of responsibilities, and measurement and control of the project."[3] This tool serves three valuable purposes:

1. It helps to further define and clarify the scope of the project.
2. Its use will help in assigning responsibility, the allocation of resources, and the overall management and control of the project.
3. It is a mechanism to use to check and double-check progress.

The first step in implementation of the WBS is to review, clarify, and communicate to all team members the scope or purpose of the project itself. The next step comes from the discussion needed to first develop the project charter and the major deliverables necessary to successfully complete the project. The key to the WBS is the determination and definition of the additional levels necessary to manage and control the entire project. The final step is to take the results back to the key stakeholders and make certain that everyone understands and is in agreement with the project work plan. Approval provided, the project can begin.

The WBS is a hierarchical look at the activities and tasks necessary to achieve project outcomes. Depending upon the presentation, there could be confusion with the practice organization chart. The WBS is not an organization chart; it is simply a representation of the project (Figure 6).

In some cases, the WBS may be presented using a spreadsheet like the one shown in Table 1. The typical hierarchy chart might only reflect columns A, B, and C. We have added the additional columns to show how the use of the tool itself can be expanded. The proj-

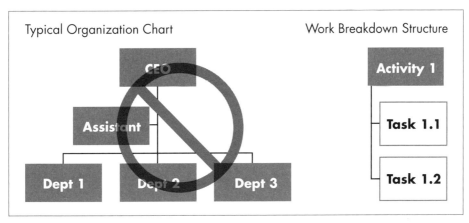

FIGURE 6. **Hierarchy chart.**

ect title is to update the practice Web site. The details on the purpose, team members, etc. are included on the project charter. This tool is added to the project charter as supplemental information. Column D reflects who is responsible for the activity and/or tasks. Column E is key in that it identifies activities or tasks that must be completed before that particular activity or task can begin. Columns F and G indicate the start and end dates, respectively, associated with each activity/task. Column H is the expected man hours budgeted to complete the project. In columns J, K, and L, the budgeted costs associated with the completion of the project are identified.

In addition to the items noted above, Table1 can be used to indicate the milestones that are reflected in the project charter; they can be further reflected here.

Once the WBS is complete, at least columns A through C, there are options to consider to assist in further managing and controlling the project. In the 1950s, the United States Navy retained Booz Allen Hamilton, Inc., to develop a model to assist in project management called the Program Evaluation and Review Technique, or PERT for short. This model was developed to help analyze the tasks involved in completing a project, paying particular attention to the time required to accomplish each task. The technique focuses on the tasks, in PERT terms "events," that are needed rather than the beginning and the end dates. The graphic presentation approach may work well for team members to understand (see Figure 7). In the example we list "acts," which are also events.

Another option to better manage from the approach of the PERT chart is to use the Critical Path Method. Figure 7 can be further refined by looking at the crucial path, which task or tasks reveal the longest individual task and/or relationship of more than one task to accomplish the project end date. Tasks B and C create one critical path equal to seven days.

TABLE 1. Work Breakdown Structure.

A	B	C	D	E	F	G	H	I	J	K	L
Project title:			Update current Web site								
					Time Frame				Costs		
#	Activity Title	Activity Components	Owner	Previous Activity	Start Date	End Date	Hours	Hourly Rate $	Payroll $	Other Costs $	Total Costs $
1.1	Secure		Joe		6/1/09	6/30/09	42	20.00	840.00		840.00
1.2		Forms									0.00
1.3		Procedure									0.00
1.4		Software								350.00	350.00
2.1	Design		Mary		6/1/09	6/30/09	18	25.00	450.00		450.00
2.2		Layout									0.00
2.3		Colors									0.00
2.4		Font									0.00
3.1	Information		Janice	2.1	6/15/09	7/15/09	27	18.00	486.00		486.00
3.2		Practice									0.00
3.3		Links									0.00
4.1	Spanish		Nancy	3.1	7/1/09	7/31/09	30	15.00	450.00		450.00
4.2		Interpretation								500.00	500.00
Total Cost											3076.00

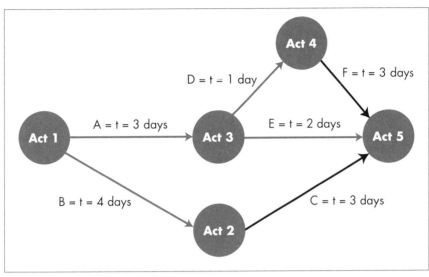

FIGURE 7. **PERT chart. t, time.**

Tasks A, D, and F also represent a critical path. Tasks A and E are not critical because they have a five-day window. Note that the activities associated with the tasks reflect milestones and that Activity 4 cannot start until Activity 3 is complete.

Yet another alternative is a Gantt chart, which is actually a spreadsheet and may be easier to create but is not a graphic. The example in Figure 8 more closely represents the concept expressed in the expanded WBS model that we discussed earlier. This example is built upon the goal of dealing with patient wait time. The plan, WBS, and Gantt chart are developed in week one. Since this is the second week of the project, the patient flow analysis is a little ahead of the anticipated time frame since the sequence indicates that the team has accomplished the percentage of activity targeted for the third week. The analysis of the scheduling process is current. The results analysis meeting and the plan preparation have yet to begin. They will begin following the completion of the patient flow analysis in week 5. Week 6 is the scheduled date for the meeting to review the results.

Project implementation

We have now reached the third phase of the life cycle. This means that the team must now perform. The details identified in the project charter dictate the time frames and resources necessary to accomplish the anticipated outcomes. The practice should have addressed and determined the appropriate deployment platform model to use in its analysis. Remember one of the goals is to standardize this process. In Chapter 5, we have detailed various de-

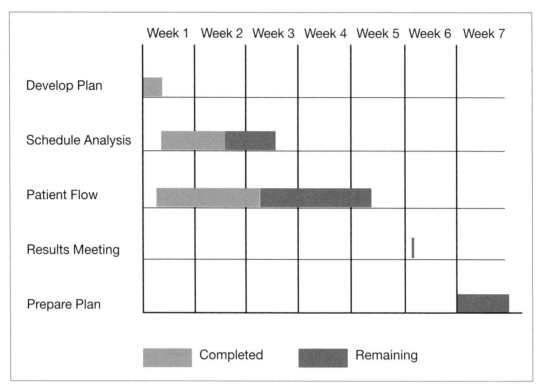

FIGURE 8. Gantt chart.

ployment options including the DMAIC, PDCS, FOCUS, IDEA, and A3, which you should refer to in making your practice determination.

All of the tables and figures used in this chapter were created either in Word, PowerPoint, or Excel. So there is no need to invest in any additional software. There are many options available to meet your overall needs and for the model that you choose to use.

However, take a look at your organization. If the choice is to follow a project management approach to achieve consistency in managing projects, then the purchase of a specific project management software program may be ideal. When purchasing, consider if there is a need for a single user or if there is a need for an enterprise (practice-wide) solution. If you need to provide access to several individuals for updates, communication, and resource utilization, the server solution for the practice may be the best way to proceed. There are many desktop as well as proprietary Web-based applications available. A quick way to gain an understanding of what is available is to go to http://en.wikipedia.org/wiki/List_of_project_management_software. One of the keys to remember is that the purchase of software does not automatically make the practice a project management-based practice. Nor does the use of a project management software package mean that the things talked about in this chapter do not have to be done.

On the contrary, it would be a waste of financial resources to purchase software without a full understanding of the project management process itself and all the tools noted throughout this book.

When it comes to implementation, there are three key areas of focus whether you use a home-grown approach or purchase software. First is simple monitoring, using the communication plan and checkpoints to ensure that things are moving according to plan. There is also the concept of control. Has someone introduced another aspect to the project? If so, is this necessary, or will it detract from the original scope? The team leader will have to step in and make the decision. If there is validity to the new task, team member, or other resource, the team leader will have to return to the project champion with a revised charter and receive approval to proceed. If the item is not considered necessary, the team leader will have to help the team regain its focus on the milestones and deliverables.

Closure

Finally is the closure. As we noted in the definition, a project is finite, it must be done. Hopefully all projects are completed successfully and the outcomes have met the mission statement! The final presentation to the stakeholders or project champion must be complete and truly representative of the initial defined scope. The recommendations for future changes must include a game plan for implementation of those changes. The process improvement plan, costs, use of resources, and appropriate metrics to measure success should be part of the recommendation.

The wait time for patients has been reduced to 10 minutes, the total time for a patient visit is now 45 minutes, the implementation of ePresribe is producing a 70% compliance rate, and so many more outcomes are noted. One of the recommendations of the initial project may be to review the project again in three or six months. It may not be the same project but the desired metric should be checked. This essentially is a milestone. If there is a feeling that the current process is working and that there is no need to revisit since improvement continues without intervention, that would be great. If not, it may be wise to reconstitute the original team. Or it may be that there are variations and the project definition needs to be revised and other staff or resources will be necessary to keep on the path to continuous improvement.

Once the project performance phase is complete, the project closure occurs. In this phase, the team members are asked to elaborate on the issues identified—those they felt were both positive and negative in the process. This information is then referred to the practice administrator and/or management team for review. The information will be used to adjust and change the practice-wide process. No project is complete without a thorough review of the process itself. Improvements made will assist in accomplishing the practice goals of standardization, which again will result in management efficiency, effective use of resources, and management of the budget for any future projects undertaken.

The end result here is that we have identified and defined a problem, utilized resources, and accomplished a targeted outcome in a systematic approach to managing a project. As you reflect on this chapter, keep in mind that there are several tools you can use and various ways that you can approach a project in your practice. The goals here are for you to identify what will work best based upon your practice mission and to develop a consistent approach to addressing the changing healthcare marketplace. You will benefit by consistency and a thorough analysis of your areas of need—either to fix or expand your practice.

Let's review the first chart in this chapter to summarize what needs to be done.

1. Project plan:
   a. Have stakeholders been identified?
   b. Does the practice (project champion) support the project?
   c. Is the charter complete?
   d. Are there other aspects of the project written such as the WBS?
2. Project definition (scope):
   a. Have the needs of the stakeholders been adequately identified?
   b. Has everyone involved agreed that the project warrants the use of resources?
3. Time involved:
   a. Have tasks been clearly defined to ensure adequate resources are available?
   b. Is the sequence correct to ensure that activities necessary to move to the milestone are in fact right? Moving to another task without completing a preceding task will cause delays and potential failure.
   c. Is the schedule right?
4. Cost involved:
   a. Is there a realistic budget in place?
   b. Are the reporting mechanisms set to ensure that costs can be monitored and controlled?
5. Quality components:
   a. Is there assurance that the project is staying within the boundaries defined as well as within the standards set for all activities in the practice?

6. Human resources:
    a. Are the rules and responsibilities clearly defined for all who are involved?
    b. Do you have the right staff with the right skills?
    c. Does the selected team have the time to devote to the project as outlined in the WBS/schedule?
    d. Is there training in place to ensure efficient use of staff?
7. Communication:
    a. Is the recorder set?
    b. Are meetings part of the schedule based upon milestones?
    c. Does the practice have an adequate intranet structure in place? Will e-mails work?
    d. Who, what, when, and how will communication work for everyone?
8. Risks:
    a. How are risks identified and defined?
    b. Which risks will affect the project?
    c. Is there a mechanism in place to measure risks and to prioritize them?
    d. Is there a plan in place to respond to risks?
9. Procurement:
    a. Are all the items necessary to complete the project already part of the practice?
    b. Will additional supplies or equipment be necessary?
    c. Will the project be able to utilize the resources targeted or will it be necessary to negotiate and therefore effectively manage relationships other than those of the actual team members?

An effective project management process will lead to significant improvements in the practice. This will have a direct impact on the key stakeholder, the patient.

References

1. BusinessDictionary.com; www.businessdictionary.com/definition/project-management.html.
2. Morris RA. *The Everything Project Management Book*, 2nd ed. Avon, MA: Adams Media; 2008.
3. Work Breakdown Structure. NetMBA.com; www.netmba.com/operations/project/wbs/.

FIVE

The TPI Toolbox

If the only tool you have is a hammer, pretty soon, everything starts to look like a nail.

EVERY INDUSTRY HAS ITS OWN TOOLBOX. For many, some of the tools are the same—things like project selection and management, or systems for measuring and benchmarking. Yet even these tools tend to be customized for not just the industry but sometimes for the specific business itself.

I am an avid cyclist. Recently, I purchased a new carbon bicycle with a carbon seat post and carbon handlebars. What I didn't know, when I made the purchase, was that pretty much every bolt and screw is subject to torque specifications. Now I already had a pretty impressive toolbox but didn't have a torque wrench. No problem, I thought, I can just buy one so I can work on the bicycle myself. What I discovered was that bicycle torque wrenches are different from, say, automobile torque wrenches as the measurement systems vary. For example, I just figured we were talking about pounds per square inch. Wrong! There are also specific metrics for Newtons per meter, inch pounds, kilogram-centimeter, etc. All have a similar definition (i.e., inch-pound is the force of one pound on an inch-long lever while Newtons per meter is the force of one Newton on a 1-meter lever), yet selecting the right tool for the job is the critical step.

In healthcare, we have the need for tools that other industries may not need and, at the same time, share many of the tools that a non-healthcare business would also require. Customizing these tools, in both structure and measurement system, is often necessary. As such, we have taken the 53 or so commonly referred to tools from the Lean Six Sigma toolbox and extracted 20 of them that seem to fit particularly well within the medical practice. Then, we customized a few of them for healthcare-specific activities. Each tool in the Total Practice Improvement (TPI) toolbox will be defined and explained; and then, to remove any confusion, we will provide the reader with an example and/or application that might be common within the practice.

Following are the 20 TPI tools that will be discussed in this chapter:

1. Process Mapping
2. Value Stream Mapping
3. Voice of the Customer
4. Kano Model
5. Critical to Quality
6. SIPOC
7. Spaghetti Diagram
8. Data Mining and Statistics
9. Ishikawa (fishbone) Diagram
10. Takt Time
11. Heijunka (load balancing)
12. Poka Yoke (mistake proofing)
13. 5S (organizational efficiency)
14. Prioritization Matrices
15. Pareto
16. Measurement System Analysis Drilldown
17. Brainstorming
18. Multi-Voting
19. Assumption Busting
20. Hypothesis Testing

PROCESS MAPPING

The first, and perhaps the most important, tool in the TPI toolbox is process mapping. First, because it precedes most other steps in the process improvement project; it is even a critical tool for project selection. But it's most important because if we did nothing else but commit to mapping each of our processes, we would realize a tremendous benefit.

What Is Process Mapping?

Most of us, at one time or another, have seen a flow chart. Sometimes flow charts are simple and represent a simple process, such as setting up a new computer. A flow chart creates a visualization of the steps involved, such as:

1. Plug in the computer.
2. Press the power switch.
3. Enter a username and password.
4. Click on the Setup button.

It might also contain a simple decision step, such as, "Were you able to set up the computer?" If the answer is "yes," well, congratulations. If the answer is "no," it might contain another step, like, "Contact your system administrator" or "Dial 1.800.WHO.CARES for technical support."

A process map provides a visual representation of a process, and it can help illustrate the tasks necessary to complete a process, the activities necessary to complete a task, and the sequence in which these events occur. Process maps also show where steps are handed off between departments. For example, at what point is the patient visit over and the billing cycle started? Properly mapped, we can *see* when the chart is handed off from clinical to billing and even the "who" involved in that step. In some cases, we will build what are called "swim lanes," which are vertical mapping lanes that show which department and/or individual is responsible for specific steps in the process.

Even though, to some, it may seem self-explanatory, many practices are reticent to get started, even when they know the mechanics involved. So why should you take the time and energy to map your processes? First (and perhaps most importantly), it is the single most efficient way to start diagnosing problems within the practice, which is the precursor to fixing and improving what you do. It helps to determine the exact cause of a problem. Root cause analysis is like the Holy Grail for many practices. You know there's a problem, and you may even know what it is; however, without getting to the root cause, you find yourself treating only the symptoms, and that doesn't support long-term or permanent solutions. Just the act of mapping a process will often reveal steps and tasks that heretofore have remained hidden from view.

Another benefit of process mapping is the training of new employees and communication with existing employees. When a process is clearly mapped, it is much easier for employees to follow the logical flow regarding steps and decision points. Process maps should be posted in associated departments and made a part of policy and procedure and training manuals. From a compliance standpoint, it helps to standardize the way things are done and communicated, reducing the risk of errors or mistakes. If you really want to provide a critical assessment of what is happening within the practice, then process mapping is the way to go. Process maps can be constructed both informally and formally, and we will look at both methods here.

Internal vs. External Impacts

Here is a mantra that can help you stay focused: "All work is part of a process." As a practical approach, there are two forces that apply: internal and external. *Internal forces* cause processes to evolve over time, including the likelihood that the practice will grow beyond its existing current state. In many cases, what began as a "good process" may erode over time, requiring a careful avoidance of traditional thinking that what was good for the organization 20 years ago is good for the organization now. That kind of thought process is not only draconian in today's competitive environment, it is counterproductive. *External forces* will drive the business model based on competitive factors and payer models; some things within your control and others not.

The issue here is that there is often a disconnect between the internal and external forces. For example, a process that is designed and operates based on operational requirements, such as those found in the billing cycle (internal force), may not be sufficient to optimize revenue under new transaction standards (external force). Because healthcare is so regulated and because (at least it seems that) physicians are bound to comply with HIPAA standard transaction rules while the payers are not, more attention is required to be paid to external forces than in many other industries.

Process Mapping Symbols

As with other tools, there are recommended ways to use them to optimize results. Figure 1 is an example of common process mapping symbols.

Before the Mapping Begins . . .

Before beginning the mapping process, it is, of course, important to select a process to map. If this is your first attempt, pick a work process that is common within the practice and one for which there are staff members that are experienced enough to assist. You might also begin with a broader overview process, such as scheduling a new visit or checking-in a patient at the front desk. Notice that these are also part of a larger work process, such as the patient visit cycle or the billing cycle.

Another salient point (and one that is often missed) is that it doesn't need to be a cycle to be "mappable." Work processes such as hiring and firing, payroll, clinical components, laboratory or imaging procedures, or even working the phones are all candidates for process mapping.

The Process Mapping Process

Even process mapping is a process, and as such, there is an order as to how it is done. Here is where the formal and the informal approach begin to diverge. In an informal approach,

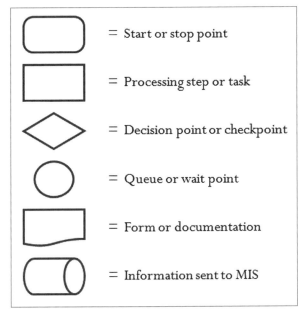

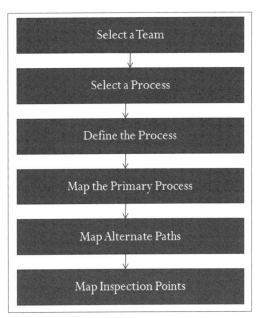

FIGURE 1. **Common process mapping symbols.** MIS, management information system.

FIGURE 2. **Overview of process mapping procedure.**

you would simply select the process, develop an "always" map, and develop the alternative map, and you are pretty much done.

From a more formal perspective (see Figure 2), usually when the map itself is part of a process improvement project rather than the purpose itself, you would first select a team and then select the process. And while it may start to sound redundant, even selecting the team is itself a process, which will be discussed later in the book. Once a process is selected, it needs to be defined; that is, its purpose, its starting point, and the expected goal. From a work perspective, you now begin to map the primary process; this is the "always" flow, meaning that everyone is subject to these steps. For example, everyone who walks into the practice must go through the check-in procedure, which may include tasks like signing a check-in sheet, validating demographics and insurance, signing a HIPAA form, etc. It wouldn't matter if this was a new patient or an existing patient, or if the patient was there to see the provider or just to have a procedure or test performed. More than likely, this would also include charting and checkout. The primary process basically defines the steps that, no matter the reason for the visit, everyone has to follow.

Once the primary path has been mapped, it is time to map the alternate paths. These are paths that some patients take while others do not. For example, a new patient may be required to fill out a new patient information package and to sign a financial release form. These steps, then, would apply only to new patients. Another example may be the reason for the visit; if the patient is there to see the provider, that is one path, but if the patient is there for a test or a procedure (i.e., laboratory screen, vaccination, injection, etc.), that would follow a totally different path. The key is this: the alternate path should diverge from the primary map (such as after check in) and merge again with the primary map (such as at checkout).

Finally, once all paths have been adequately mapped, we begin to look at inspection points along the way. This will set us up for converting our process map into a value stream map later. Inspection points are steps and tasks along the way that may be key for process improvement. These are points that have a potential for error or the risk of failure. These can be timed and for which specific personnel or departments can be assigned responsibility. Inspection points are, simply stated, places along the map that we want to "inspect" more fully for improvement potential and risk reduction.

While there is an entire chapter devoted to team development (Chapter 3), it is important to remember that in order for the mapping process to be successful, process owners need to be involved. These are the folks who walk the steps every day. Unless you are a very small practice, it would be unlikely that the administrator would understand (or even know) every step and task involved in the patient visit cycle. And it would be highly unlikely that the clinical nurse would be able to birddog the billing cycle process mapping effort.

Ironically, as we address mapping as a tool, it also has its own tools that help to optimize the work effort. Don't try your first attempt on an 8.5″ × 11″ piece of paper. Trust me on this, it's a mistake. You will want a white board and an easel and, in many cases, a blank wall and a stack of sticky-backed notepads. The white board is great for being able to visualize your thoughts and make corrections on the fly. The bigger the board the better, and the more notes you write the better. Have a digital camera with you, and photograph your work before you erase it. This is also a great reason to have a flip chart—it gives you a running record of your creative work. Each time you fill a sheet, take it off the pad and tape it to the wall. The sticky notepaper is one of the best ways I know to begin the mapping process. Have one or two people as recorders; they will write down the steps that are called out by the team (if there is a team) and put them on the white board or the wall. These are then later organized into "always," "sometimes," and "rarely" groups for mapping primary and alternative paths.

Defining the Process

From the high point, defining the process to map may seem pretty simple; pick a process, any process. But there is a difference between "selecting" the process to map and "defining" the process to map. In fact, defining the process comes *after* selection. The most important task here is to determine to whom the process is focused. In essence, who are the customers? If we aren't engaging in process improvement to make life better for our customers, then I haven't done a very good job so far in this book.

One constraint we face is that, in healthcare, the word "customer" sounds and feels foreign. After all, we don't have customers, we have patients. *Webster's* dictionary defines the word *customer* in this simple way: someone who pays for a product or a service. Hmmm. In our business, the person or entity that actually pays for the service often involves a multitude, and some would argue that, based on this definition, it is *not* the patient (or at least, not only the patient). But the fact is, patients pay for their healthcare either through co-pays, direct pay, premiums, payroll deductions, and/or taxes. And they aren't the only ones. The payers pay (although not as often, timely, or accurately as they should). The patients' employer pays. And if you look at the non-dollar component involved, even the practice's staff could be considered a customer. Now, not every customer can always be considered with each mapping project; however, if there isn't a customer involved, then the value of the project is significantly reduced.

Once the customer(s) has/have been identified, spend a few moments getting to understand their requirements. There are three primary components to the consumer model: quality, speed, and value. The old joke is, pick any two. So if you want quality and speed, you sacrifice value; if you want value and speed, you sacrifice quality; and if you want value and quality, you sacrifice speed. It even sounds like it makes sense! In every case, however, one or more of these requirements fit the customers' needs.

The final step is to define the starting and finishing points in the map. This is the first step and the last. For example, when hiring a new employee, the process may begin with writing the job description or placing an ad, or, in some cases, you may define the starting point as the interview. The final step could be when the employee is hired, or, for some practices, it may extend to the end of the probation period. For a patient visit, you could define the start as when the appointment is made, or, for some practices, it could start when the patient checks in. In one practice I worked with, the start was the appointment time and didn't consider whether the patient was early or late. The end of the map could be when the patient checks out, or, alternatively, after the chart has been completed and submitted for billing.

Building the Process Map

I often refer to this as the Zen of process mapping. The key here is to "be the thing" that is to be mapped. Interestingly, very few administrators I have met have ever actually gone through the patient visit cycle from start to finish. When I work with a practice on process improvement, my first action step is to call the practice, schedule an appointment, and go through the entire visit cycle. I carry with me a notepad, pencil, and a stopwatch, and I record (and time) every step and task that occurs. My experience is this: in the overwhelming majority of cases, when I compare my list to the initial process map the practice suggests, I have 20% to 30% more steps/tasks than the practice listed in its first mapping attempt. Be the thing! If it's a patient visit, then be the patient. If it's the billing cycle, then be the claim. If it's a hiring issue, be the resume or the candidate. Be the thing!

Once the start and finish points have been established, trace the process from beginning to end, making sure to separate the "always" from the "sometimes" steps. This is where the sticky notes come in. Whether you have a team or you are the team, using brainstorming techniques (defined later), write down every single step that you (or your team) can think of that is a part of the process. Every step, irrespective of whether it happens always, sometimes, or rarely, is still part of the process. Write each step on a sticky note, and stick it to a wall or a white board (make sure you have a large white board).

Once you have exhausted this effort (or just the team members!), begin to organize the notes on the wall into three columns. In the left column, put the start and finish steps (top and bottom respectively) along with the "always" steps in order of occurrence, again from top to bottom. In the next column (to the right), put the "sometimes" steps for each of the collateral or alternate paths. Some of these, such as laboratory studies, will actually become their own process maps. Finally, in the far right column, put those steps that occur rarely. Look for rework loops as you go through this. A rework loop is a cyclical process that occurs as a result of mistakes or potential mistakes that occur often—for example, having to recertify a procedure or reverify insurance or recollect demographic information from a patient. The idea is to stay as high-level as possible so those steps that look like they will form their own processes should be included as steps here and put in queue for a later process mapping project.

Map the Primary Process First

As discussed, the primary process includes the basic steps necessary to produce the output. Remember, these are the steps that everyone goes though in order to be satisfied that the process has been completed. Figure 3 shows some examples:

Note that in the patient visit, every patient has to check in, wait in the waiting room, see the provider, and check out. This isn't to say that there aren't other steps, such as a test or procedure, but the point is that not *every* patient has to go through those steps. If the patient is

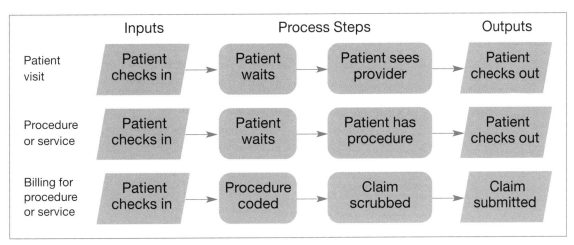

FIGURE 3. **Examples of primary processes.**

there for a procedure or service only, then the patient still checks in, waits, and checks out, as well as having the procedure or service or test performed. Regarding the billing process, irrespective of the reason for the visit, each one is subject to a chart review, assignment of ICD-9 and/or HCPCS code(s), claim scrubbing (this may not occur in all practices, but for this practice, it occurs prior to submitting every claim), and then the claim submission.

Examples

Patient Visit for Appointment with the Provider

First, map the primary path. Start with the "always" process steps, such as:

- The patient checks in (starting point).
- The patient waits in the waiting room.
- The patient is escorted by someone to the exam room.
- The patient sees the provider.
- The encounter is documented and then coded.
- The patient checks out.

The assumption is that all patients will experience at least these steps.

Decision Points

Many of the alternate paths that will ultimately be a part of the final map are determined based on what are called decision points. Decision points are pretty self-explanatory in that they simply represent a point on the map that requires a decision in order to continue. In standard parlance, decision points are represented as diamonds. Decision points can be

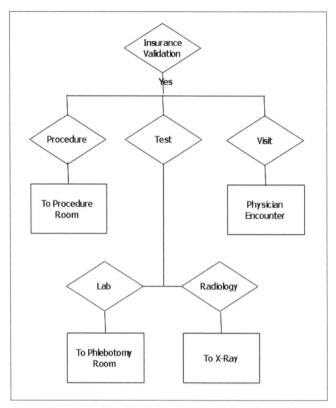

FIGURE 4. Decision points.

mapped in a number of ways, such as simple Yes or No paths. For example, in the patient visit, we may want to know the following:

- Is this a new or established patient?
- Were we able to validate insurance?
- Is the patient there for a procedure/test or to see the provider?

In the above examples, each decision point includes an additional branch for each Yes or No answer.

Decision points can also be more complex than just simple Yes or No responses. In a map with multiple-type decision points, each diamond may create its own branch. For example, instead of setting up several Yes/No paths for the reason for the visit (Procedure? No. Test? No. Visit? Yes.), you may base the alternate paths on selecting the response in a more parallel fashion. For example, you may have three diamonds, each with only one response; Yes.

In the example shown in Figure 4, you can see that a different branch is established for each Yes response to the reason for the visit. You see this again when the positive response to "Test" results in additional decision points; is the test a laboratory or a radiology procedure?

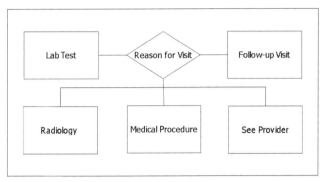

FIGURE 5.   One decision point results in several paths.

You can also see a situation in which one decision point results in several paths based on a multiple-choice response, as in the example shown in Figure 5.

In this case, each may either be dependent or independent of the other paths, and each may require its own process map.

Figure 6 is an example of a process map for a typical billing cycle.

Maps can also be developed as cross functional. In a cross-functional map, the process flow is similar, only it may be categorized by phase or even by department. The idea is to maintain the logical flow as the phases should interrelate to process responsibilities. This type of map is more complex to design and normally requires a cross-functional team in order to be completed accurately. Figure 7 is an example of a simple cross-functional map.

Some process maps take on far more complex modeling than what we have discussed here, such as what you see in Figure 7; these are known as swim lanes. Some maps follow totally different designs, such as circular or non-linear maps. While these have applications in manufacturing and some service industries, they have limited functionality within the medical practice.

Inspection Points

The final step is to identify inspection points. These are steps and/or tasks in the map that are identified as candidates for critical inspections. The purpose is to identify potential errors before they reach the consumer. For example, at check in, the patient may arrive late, be unprepared to pay the co-pay for the visit, or may not have current insurance information. At check out, you may discover that the provider didn't document adequately to assign a code, and, therefore, patient payment responsibility may not be able to be assessed. In the billing process, failure to properly modify a procedure may results in a claim rejection or a denial. This step falls just short of creating the value stream map in that no data are

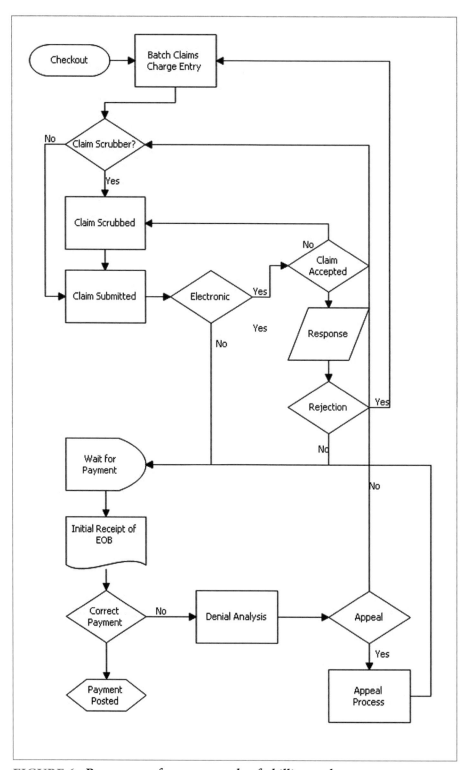

FIGURE 6. Process map for one example of a billing cycle.

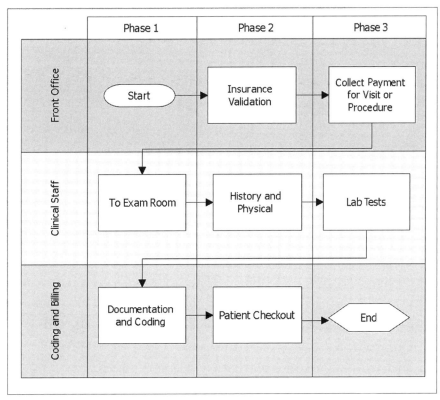

FIGURE 7. **Cross-functional process map.**

collected. Identifying these steps accurately will, however, feed the next phase, which is, in fact, value stream mapping.

VALUE STREAM MAPPING

If you do what you've always done, you'll get what you've always gotten.

—Anthony Robbins

Value stream mapping (VSM) picks up from the process mapping step and starts as a paper-and-pencil tool that helps you to see and understand the flow of object, patients, materials, supplies, and information as a product (patient) or service (procedure) makes its way through the value stream.

VSM differs from process mapping in four ways:

1. It gathers and displays a far broader range of information than a typical process map.
2. It tends to be more specific than process maps.

3. It tends to be used at a broader level (i.e., from inventory to accounting to clinical).

4. It tends to be used to identify where to focus future projects, subprojects, and/or Kaizen events.

A value stream map takes into account not only the activity of the procedure/service, but the management and information systems that support the basic process. This is especially helpful when working to reduce cycle time, because you gain insight into the decision-making flow in addition to the process flow. In VSM, the basic idea is to first map your process, then map the information flow that enables the process to occur.

Four Phases of Value Stream Mapping

There are four distinct phases in VSM. Phase 1 involves mapping the process; and by the time you get here, this should already have been done. Phase 2 involves the process of data mining and data collection. Much of these data are collected from what we refer to here as a "data box." As the data box is completed (meaning that data and information are entered into the appropriate fields), it is often displayed on the map itself, adding to the visual power of the map. Phase 3 involves analyzing the data, and this involves both data mining and statistical analyses, both of which are discussed later in this chapter. It is from the analysis that you create the work product, and from the work product that you conduct your root cause analyses, which are used to identify not on the "what" but the "where" and "why" of problems. Finally, in phase 4, you use the information and the visual display to create solutions to the problems discovered during the VSM step.

Phase 1: Map the Process

Not to belabor the steps, you should have come to the VSM step with your process map completed, approved, and in hand.

Figure 8 is an example of a process map that will be used for VSM. Note the conventions used to identify inspection points.

Phase 2: Data Collection

In phase 2, you want to begin to collect data that will be used in your assessment of each step in the process. First and foremost, you want to know, ahead of time, what data you need (or want) versus what data you can actually collect. For example, you may want to analyze denials as part of the revenue cycle, but if your practice management system (PMS) doesn't record this information from the 835s (the electronic equivalent of the CMS 1500 billing form), it is unlikely you will have access to either rates or reasons. In

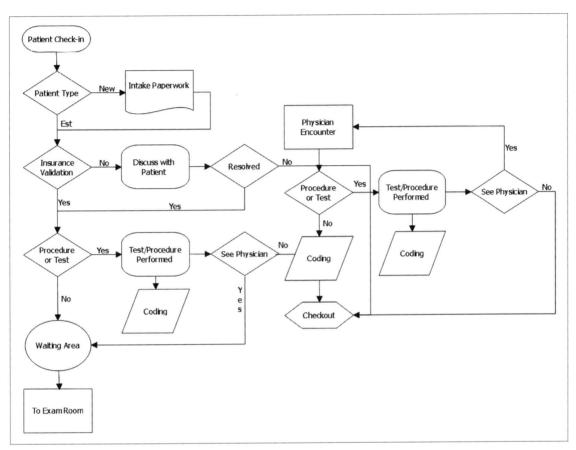

FIGURE 8. **Patient visit cycle.**

some (and sometimes many) cases, you will need to depend on primary research in order to access the needed data. Primary research usually involves designing an experiment, such as a method to obtain the number of minutes (or seconds or hours) a step requires for completion. This is particularly important when looking at cyclical processes, such as the patient visit or the billing cycle.

Sometimes, you may be able to access existing studies that pertain to data you would like to review. For example, there is a great study that estimates the average rate of disagreement for E/M code categories amongst coding professionals[1]; or another study released in October of 2007 that deals with the profitability of uninsured vs. insured patients.[2] You may have had a consultant or staff person conduct a study or analysis of some internal clinical or operational process in the past. Don't disregard these data as they can be used to help design a future study; assist with benchmarking a process or a step; or, in some cases, even serve as a proxy for data you may want to collect but for whatever reason, are not able to do so.

Sometimes, you will need outside assistance to ensure accurate and timely data collection. Look for specialists within your organization, such as your information technology department (if you have one) or a staff member that specializes in that particular area. The most important task in this step is to have a written data collection plan. This should include, in addition to the "what," the "who," 'how," and "when" steps. In fact, I have often seen a separate process map developed for data collection as it is, in its own right, a process.

The Data Box.   Earlier, I referred to the data box and the importance of standardizing this for your practice. The data box is actually a checklist, of sorts, that specifies the type of data that are commonly required in order to build a VSM.

For our purposes here, the data box consists of the following items:

- Who does it;
- How many people it takes;
- Cycle time for the task;
- Average daily requirement (daily demand rate [DDR]);
- Delay time prior to the task;
- Process step details;
- Average delay before this step occurs;
- Total units waiting (claims, patients, charts, etc.);
- Top three rework issues;
- Top three risks; and
- Artifacts (screen captures, forms, traceable documents, etc.).

Let's look at these one at a time.

Who does it.   Fairly self explanatory, the idea here is to assign responsibility for the step or task to a particular person, persons, or department. For example, who conducts simple lab studies? Is it the nurse, is it the provider, or does the practice employ lab technicians? Some tasks may be shared, such as in clinical steps or in the coding and/or billing steps. If this is the case, it may be a good idea to specify the percent of responsibility. For example, when the patient is seen by the provider, 75% of the responsibility may be assigned to the provider and 25% to the clinical assistant who may assist with an exam.

How many people it takes.   Different from above, we want to identify the number of staff persons that touch that step. For example, when looking at the hiring process, it may involve the HR director, the department head, and the administrator—all sharing in the responsibility for recommending for or against the hire.

Cycle time for the task. As a direct measurement, how long does it take for the task to be completed? This isn't necessarily asking for the "average" time at this point as that is normally calculated in the analysis step. Here, you want the actual time for that specific event. If you were designing an experiment to measure the average time a patient spends in the waiting room, you would determine, in advance, how many patients you wanted to sample, and the metric in this field of the data box would represent the actual time for the patient being studied. In the analysis step, you would use all of the data from all of the patients (samples) to calculate the average waiting time.

DDR. The DDR is just the average daily requirement to meet this step. It could be the number of patients per day, claims per hour, or appeals per week.

Process step details. Here, you want to take the process step itself and break it down into the individual required tasks. For example, in the check-out step, the tasks might include coding the visit (or procedure), passing this along to the check-out person, collecting any payment from the patient, scheduling the next appointment, etc.

Delay time prior to the task. This metric is particularly important when collecting data for cyclical processes. For example, during the patient encounter with the provider, there may be a period of time that occurs between when the patient is left in the exam room and the provider actually sees the patient (often times referred to as "the second waiting room").

Total units waiting. This can be patients (as in the number waiting in the waiting room), number of charts to be filed, or number of claims to be reviewed. This may also be the number of lab tests in the queue or even the number of resumes to be reviewed.

Top three rework issues. This may well be the most important step regarding process improvement. Not to minimize the other fields in the data box, the top three rework issues tie directly to the cost of doing business. These are issues that, when done incorrectly or are error prone due to circumstances outside of the practice's control (such as payer schemes and games), result in the necessity to redo (or rework) the step in the process. For example, regarding a laboratory test, failure to meet medical necessity might require resubmission of the claim, or failure to calibrate the equipment may result in the need to redo the test.

Top three risks. This field in the data box goes directly to the heart of consequences due to errors, mistakes, and other issues that create risk in the practice. For example, not ensuring that the patient has signed the financial responsibility form could lead to a situation in which you can't collect your co-pay at the time of visit. Reporting blood work for the wrong patient could result in inappropriate treatment and even harm to the patient. Language barriers could prevent the practice from getting an accurate history, including information about drug allergies.

Artifacts. Artifacts are items that are necessary for a task to take place. For example, they could include an encounter form or super bill, the lab requisition document, or a screen capture from the PMS or electronic medical record (EMR) system. Artifacts are sometimes collateral and sometimes directly influence the process efficiency, such as duplicate forms in a new patient intake package.

Here is an example of a patient check-in:

- Who does this?
  — Front-office staff
- How many people does it take?
  — One person (at a time)
- Cycle time for the task
  — From 3 to 15 minutes, depending on risk factors
  — Consider stratification of data points
    • New patient, established patient, referral type, etc.
- DDR
  — 78 patients per day for check in
    • Calculate total time each day (i.e., 9 min $\times$ 78 = 702 min = 11.7 hrs/day)
    • Translates to ~1.5 FTE dedicated staff person
- Delay time prior to the task (how long does it take between the end of the last task and the beginning of this task?)
- Process step details
  1. Initiate paperwork (new patient?).
     a. HIPAA form
     b. Sign financial policy form
     c. Any waivers (i.e., Advance Beneficiary Notice if appropriate)
     d. Referral and pre-authorization verification
  2. Verify patient using ID (i.e., driver's license).
  3. Verify insurance (or reverify).
  4. Make sure all forms are complete and in the package.
  5. Collect co-pay (if applicable).
  6. Notify clinical staff that patient has arrived.
- Average delay before this step occurs
  — None (this is the first step), or
  — Time from appointment to visit (important metric)

- Number of patients waiting
  — 12 in queue (waiting room)
- Top three quality or rework issues
  — Incorrect insurance information (i.e., certification or guarantor)
  — Insurance plan has changed
  — Demographics incorrect
- Top three risk factors
  — Language barrier
  — Inability to collect co-pay in advance
  — Patient late or no-show
- Artifacts
  — New patient package
  — Financial responsibility form
  — Sign-in log
  — Screen capture from PMS scheduling program

Remember, the VSM, like the process map, can be formal or informal, and there are many different models available to review and/or follow.

Phase 3: Analyze the Data

The first step in the data analysis phase is to separate useful data from stuff that is just fun to know. For example, knowing how long a patient waits in the waiting room may be important but knowing which magazines (if any) or what channels (if any) the patient looks at may not. It used to be, years ago, we couldn't get enough data. Today, the problem is often that we get too much, and in this case, more is not necessarily better. As mentioned prior, having a data collection plan is a good way to prevent this potential bottleneck from occurring. In common parlance, it is referred to as "analysis paralysis." There are actually two components to phase 3; one involves data analysis, and the other involves statistical analysis.

Data analysis allows you to get an overview of process steps, such as trends, comparative benchmarks, etc. Statistical analysis allows you to determine the significance of what you are seeing. For example, you may be trying to determine whether one physician in the practice is more productive or works harder (two distinctly different metrics) than the other physicians. A data analysis will give you, in this case, the number of work RVUs, allowing you to see the difference among providers or the difference between a provider and a control group. Statistical analysis will help you to understand if the differences you are seeing are significant or just the results of noise, or common variability. In this example, you might find provider 1 reporting an average of 460 work RVUs per month while provider 2 reports 480 work RVUs per month. You got this result by graphing the monthly work RVUs for the past year and looking at trending and averaging the annual results. Anecdotally, you might say that provider 2 reports more work RVUs than provider 1, which he or she clearly does based on your data analysis. But, statistically speaking, is there really a difference between 460 and 480 work RVUs? The answer is, maybe and maybe not. From the statistical point of view, you might calculate the 95% confidence interval for each of the doctors and find out that the values intersect at some point. In this case, it would mean that the difference between the two (the 20 work RVUs per month) is nothing more than noise—the common variability that you expect to see as a result of normal practice variation.

Regarding the trends, a data analysis might show a trend that goes up, goes down, or vacillates during the data period, and we might hypothesize the impact of what we see. Statistics, however, would measure the trends and report with a high degree of certainty as to whether there really was a trend or not. Understanding statistics is bigger than what we can cover here; however, in nearly every other industry, mid- to upper-level management has at least a basic understanding of business statistics, and it shouldn't be any different in a medical practice.

The key is to look for variability in the data, and then test the significance using statistical methods. The fact is, people don't notice averages; they notice variability. When you drive to work, I would be willing to bet that you notice far less often the times that it takes you about an average amount of minutes (or hours) to get there than the times when it takes you twice as long for the same trip. In a crowd of people, we would be much less likely to notice folks who are an "average" height as opposed to someone that is very tall (say 6′10″) or very short. In a crowded room, we would be less likely to notice conversations that go on in our own (or a common) language as opposed to one that was conducted in a language we had never heard.

When analyzing data, the same is true. If you graphed denials reported each week as a percent of total claims filed, you would be much more likely to notice a spike of 8.4% than the average denial rate of 3.5%. The real gold is found in variability, and the great news is that, when the proper visual techniques are used, variability is very easy to see. The other key is accountability. When variability is discovered, someone within the organization should be able to explain, in understandable and clear language, the reason for the variation. For example, if denials did spike one week to 8.4%, someone within the practice should be able to tell you why. If no one can do this, then you have found an area that may likely require process improvement.

Figure 9 illustrates an analysis of cycle time for an established patient visit.

For the example shown in Figure 9, the total visit cycle time was 106.7 minutes, or 1.8 hours. Visual representations are very important for effective communication of your results. Figure 10 shows both the individual time for each step as well as the cumulative time as the steps progress.

The illustration in Figure 11 defines statistics for each of the crucial steps in a clinical process as well as the variation calculated for a given set of sample data. This VSM example even gives the goal in number of minutes as well as the percentage of time the goal was met.

Risks and Errors. In addition to more commonly accepted data, as mentioned before, we want to be able to identify the risk of mistakes and errors and the subsequent risk that may result from them. During the patient check-in, these may include such things as the patient being

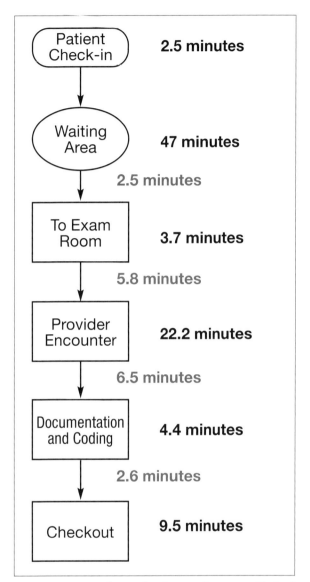

FIGURE 9. Analysis of cycle time for an established patient visit. Numbers in teal represent the time between steps.

late, confusion over the appointment time, and even the reason for the visit. In fact, as we often see, the patient may have misstated or outright lied about the chief complaint such that what the patient said when the appointment was made is totally different from what the patient says when he or she sees the provider. Maybe the patient can't properly complete the intake paperwork or he or she may owe money from a prior visit (or co-pay for this visit) and either have forgotten a method of payment or simply don't have the means to

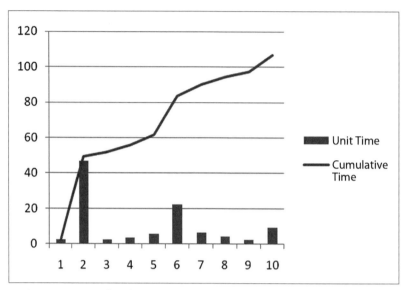

FIGURE 10. Individual time for each step as well as the cumulative time as the steps progress.

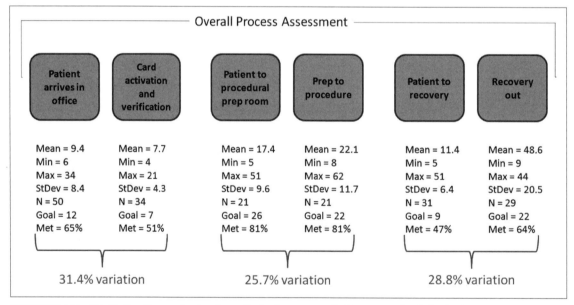

FIGURE 11. Statistics for each step in a clinical process. St Dev, standard deviation.

pay at that time. I have seen situations where the patient chart is still out from the prior visit and can't be located.

There are lots of opportunities for these kinds of issues during the insurance validation step of the patient visit. If validation is done via the telephone directly with the payer,

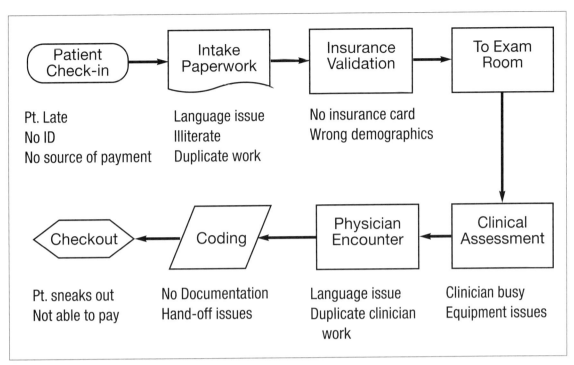

FIGURE 12. **Potential error points that may require rework.**

it may take a long time for someone to give you the information you need. In some cases, it may take so long you just give up, opening the door for a denial of payment at a later date. The payer could give the wrong information or, as has been often reported to us, the payer might just lie. Maybe the patient has incorrect demographic information or, as mentioned before, the patient may not have the ability to pay. In each of these examples, there is a subsequent risk that the practice faces. It could be the cost of rework or the loss of revenue from a claim that won't get paid. It could be a clinical issue such as with the case of a patient that lies, or one that is illiterate, or where a language barrier prevents completion of documentation. You may have to make a decision whether to see a patient that refuses to pay, and this requires an understanding of the laws that govern your practice.

Often, the only risk from errors and mistakes is rework; but remember, when you can't cut costs any further than you have and you realize little control over revenue, the only way to maintain and/or increase profitability is through increasing efficiency. And that translates to reducing waste and cycle times. Rework is the antithesis to both. Figure 12 is a VSM that shows errors that would require rework for the practice.

By incorporating data analysis and statistics, you begin to quantify even what appear to be only nominal data points, as shown in Figure 13.

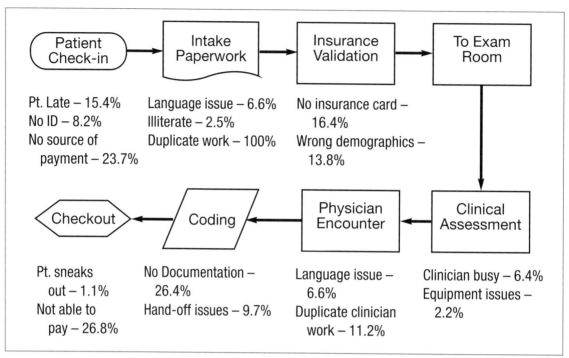

FIGURE 13. Applying data analysis and statistics to data points.

Phase 4: Improve the Process

At first, this seems a bit flip, similar to Nancy Reagan's "Just Say No" solution for fighting drug abuse in the United States. That worked fine for people not addicted to drugs, but ask a heroin addict his or her opinion of that strategy, and you would likely get a different response.

In any case, once you have been able to map the process, collect the data, and conduct your analysis, it starts to feel like fixing things is more doable than overwhelming. I have always been amazed at some of the annual conferences I attend where the same people are complaining about the same problems year after year after year. Why is it that if they know what the problem is, they don't just fix it so they can find something different to complain about the next year? It is because they have not taken the time to formalize the steps that we have discussed heretofore.

Think about it. If your car was making a strange noise and the consequence was a reduction in gas mileage and you were able to determine the cause of the problem, what is the likelihood that you would get it fixed (assuming you could afford to fix it)? I would estimate it would be pretty high. What we have discussed so far is nothing

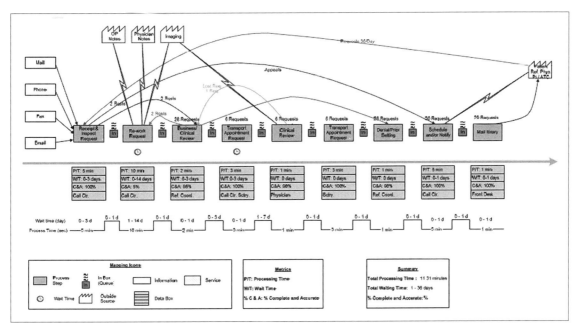

FIGURE 14. Current-state process map.

more than differential diagnosis for the practice and that should be familiar to just about everyone in our field.

You use the information from the VSM steps and analysis phase specifically to do a root cause analysis of the issues discovered. For each problem or potential problem (a step that may not be a problem now but has a risk of being a problem in the future), you create a contingency plan, "What will we do if . . . ?" Once you have discussed, tested, and recommended the improvements, you create a future-state process map. This is nothing more than the current-state process map with the new steps added or old steps removed. It should include specific goals for each step as well as contingency plans for each.

Figures 14 and 15 are examples I found for a current-state map (Figure 14) converted into a future-state map (Figure 15).

VSM Challenges in the Medical Practice

The medical practice faces some unique challenges when it comes to creating the value stream map. This is particularly true when compared with industries such as manufacturing or even some sectors in service industries. For one, the speed of change in medicine is usually slower. I read a study a while ago that claimed it took upwards of 15 years for a new medical or surgical technique, once published, to reach most medical practices. In addi-

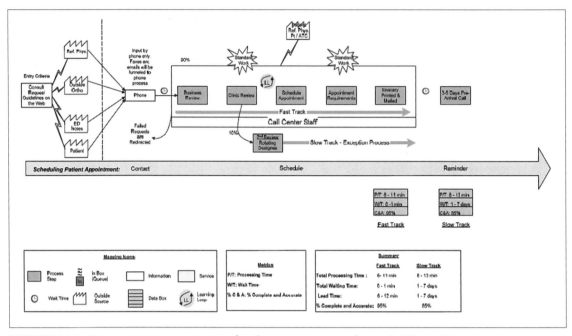

FIGURE 15. Future-state process map for the same process shown in Figure 14.

tion, policies are usually well established (or should we say that tradition is often well en-
trenched), and politics gets in the way. The medical practice is a classical example of too many
cooks . . . Because our industry is very new to business technology (look at our poor progress
regarding EMRs), it is often more difficult to establish the metrics needed to measure and
analyze processes and obtain results. And even though it is sometimes easy to see what
needs fixing (the coder comes in at 10:00 a.m. and leaves at 2:00 p.m.), it normally takes
longer to achieve results. Last, but certainly not least, establishing the true cost of quality
and the cost of the process is much more difficult than in other industries.

VOICE OF THE CUSTOMER

*The best way to understand your customer is to become your
customer and walk a mile in their shoes.*

—IAN D. LITTMAN

I wonder how often we in healthcare take a look at how satisfied our customers are with
the care that we provide. Healthcare is, after all, a service industry; and more than most, it
delivers personal service in the form of healthcare to its patients. A 2005 Forrester research
survey[3] showed that 96% of senior executives believed that improving customer satisfac-

tion was either "critical" or "very critical" to their future plans and success. Yet, in that same survey, the majority of those folks surveyed admitted that they were delivering "sub-par experiences to the customer." In most other industries, the customer is pretty easy to identify; but in healthcare, because of the pervasiveness of insurance and the complexity of payer models, it is often difficult to identify who, in reality, constitutes the customer. The critical question for us, however, is this: if we can identify the customer, do we really care about his or her experience? Let's move forward with that question in mind.

Understanding the Customer

The first step in understanding your customer is to define your customer, and, as noted above, this is sometimes particularly difficult in healthcare. The customer, for most purposes, is the recipient of the product or service. Note that, in our industry, the recipient of the service is often different from the person paying for the service, and in some instances, different from the person paying for the service *and* the person receiving the service. Confused? Join the club!

In pediatrics, for example, it is often the parent (or parents) that is the customer rather than the patient. And in most cases, except for the uninsured, it is the payer that is included as the customer; even though the payer is not the recipient, it is, in fact, paying for the service.

From the perspective of process improvement and true voice of the customer (VOC) parlance, it would be a mistake not to also consider the staff (including the providers) as customers. In many cases, it will also include vendors, such as PMS and EMR companies; lab and other outpatient providers; hospitals; and pretty much anyone else who touches the services provided to the patient.

Having defined the customer (hopefully!), it is important to get a better understanding of the entity to whom we are referring. One step is to understand the difference between a need and a requirement. A need establishes the relationship and is subject to the specific service or procedure. For example, when I fly, my defined *need* is to walk off the plane (meaning we land safely). For a patient, the need might be a proper diagnosis and treatment or to wake up after a surgical procedure. For a payer, the need might be a properly completed claim or accompanying documentation. This is how the need establishes the basis for the relationship.

The requirement differs in that, rather than establishing the relationship, it defines customer satisfaction. Back to the flying example: my need is to get off the plane safely and without injury. My requirement is to land somewhere near my original destination at somewhere near the expected time. For a patient, while the need is a proper diagnosis and treatment, a requirement might be to be seen within a reasonable amount of time—say 30 minutes. For the payer, while a clean claim is a need for proper payment, a requirement might be electronic submission (837) rather than a paper claim (CMS-1500).

Hearing the Voice of the Customer

Assuming that you really do care about the customers and what they think, you have to put forth some effort, then, to find out what they think (or for some, how they feel). It is quite useless to design a customer-oriented model without getting input from the customers. I believe this is why so many PMS programs, for example, are not user-friendly; they were designed by programmers without getting input from the office staff. I asked a friend of mine once, rather rhetorically, why, with the newer cars, I couldn't even change may own sparkplugs, and his response was because cars were designed by engineers, not mechanics.

In order to determine the needs and requirements of your customers, you need to ask them their opinion, and there are six primary methods to accomplish this:

1. Interviews
2. Focus groups
3. Market research
4. Surveys
5. Personal observation
6. Customer complaints

For each method, you want to examine the resources required against the level of accuracy and detail you wish to attain. In order to validate your results, you need to employ more than one of these methods.

Interviews

Interviews involve either one-on-one contact with the customer (or potential customer) or, as with a focus group, a number of customers at the same time.

Pros. There is little more that is of greater value in a market research study than the ability to personally observe the subject(s). Personal observation is, at times, more important than the responses themselves, as a trained observer can often tell if individuals are being honest, if they are uncomfortable with the question, if they are guessing, or if they are engaged in any other activity that would threaten to invalidate their results. Body language and eye movements can be critical indicators regarding the validity of the information you are receiving. This method also offers a high degree of flexibility in that you can change the questions or the direction of the interview on the fly based on the responses (or lack of responses) you are getting from the subject. And when a question invokes a response that, in many cases, includes more information than anticipated, you can drill-down to a greater level of detail simply by asking more questions.

Cons. Personal interviews are often far more expensive when you consider the time required to obtain information from one respondent. A properly conducted interview can take several hours to complete, depending on the level of granularity required. In many cases, personal interviews are conducted because there is a high level of criticality surrounding the project or process being considered, and if several people are involved in the decision process, the time and expense involved can increase precipitously. For example, the decision sought may include the purchase of an expensive piece of imaging equipment or an EMR system, or perhaps the practice is looking to hire a specialist in some competitive area like hand surgery or oncology. Any one of these may place a great deal of money at risk, and therefore, one cannot afford to obtain bad or wrong information from the respondents, particularly if their responses determine the direction or flow of the project. In these cases, it may be necessary to hire someone trained in conducting these types of interviews, such as a market researcher or facilitator, which adds to the cost of the interview. Finally, as evident from this discussion, for all the time, effort, and resources committed, the sample size will ultimately be quite small—from only one person to a maximum of a handful.

Focus Groups

As with interviews, a focus group is a type of qualitative research model that, rather than looking to assess responses as a percent of some target, looks to obtain opinions and attitudes that are later used to develop a more quantitative study. Focus groups are normally employed to assist a company with ideas on new products and services or ways to improve existing ones. The key feature of a focus group is the ability to obtain opinions from potential customers about product and service ideas and to observe individuals within the dynamics of a group setting. Regarding a medical practice, a focus group may be desirable when considering adding new services, such as in the area of cosmetic surgery or weight loss. It could also involve a group of existing patients to get their opinion on a new location for an office or an administrative decision, such as payment options, that could affect a patient's loyalty to the practice itself.

Pros. As with the interview, one of the most important features of a focus group is the ability to personally observe the respondents; both as individuals and as members of a group. It is important to be able to assess whether a particular person's answer truly represents his or her own opinion or whether the individual simply acquiesces to the dynamics of the group. Unlike anonymous-type research models, such as with surveys, personal observation is a positive feature of this technique. From a cost perspective, it also allows you to "interview" more than one person at a time. If, for example, you are looking to add a new service to the practice, you can get simultaneous opinions on the likelihood of using the service and the willingness to pay out-of-pocket from up to a dozen people at the same time. And the answers and concerns expressed during the meeting are most often used to create a quantitative study (such as a survey) that is used to obtain similar information from a much larger audience.

Cons. One of the greatest risks involved with focus groups is the effect that group dynamics has on an individual. People who in a one-on-one interview may have no problem expressing their own opinions may fee stifled in a group setting. As a result, you end up with "group think" rather than true individual thoughts and ideas. In some cases, this is the desired effect, such as when studying the influence a group may have on an individual's responses. Most of the time, however, suppression of someone's true opinion negates the value of having a focus group in the first place. Focus groups can also be expensive in that the participants need to be properly vetted, similar to that of a jury. It is important that those involved in the group are part of the target market being sought. In its simplest sense, you wouldn't want a male involved in a group opining on the value of services specifically directed toward women, or childless adults considering additional products and services that are pediatric in nature. More so than with interviews, because of the "group therapy" nature of a focus group, it is important to have one or more professional facilitators involved with the project. This will add to the cost of the effort; however, the quality of the outcomes can often be affected by the quality of the facilitator(s).

Market Research

Market research is a broad-stroke model that can be inclusive of a number of designs and techniques. The two areas of market research are primary and secondary. Primary research involves the design of a new experiment, test or other approach, such as the interviews and focus groups mentioned above. It also includes the design of survey instruments and conducting a large mailing of those surveys, for example. Secondary research involves the analysis of existing studies, such as that found with a meta analysis. Secondary research has the advantages of being less expensive and piggy-backing onto someone else's work. It also has the disadvantage of compromise in that, it most cases, the prior work is not specific for your needs.

Pros. Market research allows for a much larger sample of respondents and therefore quickly becomes quantitative in nature. This is important when you are looking to see what percent of a given population would be willing to pay for a given product or service as opposed to how that product or service would be designed or marketed (as discovered in a focus group). Having a larger sample allows for the development of critical statistical models, such as confidence intervals, standard deviations, and other measurements of central tendency and variability. These are important tools of inferential statistics, as our goal is often to take the data from our study and predict the behavior for a much larger audience of people. For example, we may have discovered that 15% of our given target market would be somewhat or very likely to spend the desired amount of a particular service the practice is planning to offer. From a planning perspective, we want to be able to predict, with 95% confidence, the number of people that would use the service for a broader geographic market. In this case, if our 95% confidence interval were 12% to 18%, I could predict, with 95% confidence, that the actual number of potential patients, in a population of 100,000, would be somewhere between 12,000 and 18,000; numbers critical for strategic and logistical planning. The other benefit to this type of research is that it is normally outsourced. You pay a professional market research firm to develop and conduct the study, and you just interpret the results.

Cons. The first negative is related to the last positive; outsourcing. You need to accept the fact that, in most outsourced circumstances, you will lose control of the design and research for the study; that is why you are paying someone else. Obviously, there is an expectation that whoever is in charge of the project will properly screen the market research firms; but in any case, you add a degree of uncertainty to the results that cannot be determined by statistical calculations. This is a garbage in-garbage out model (GIGO) and requires time and effort to pick the right firm. As a result of the vetting process and the potential size of the study, it can be expensive and this needs to be considered as a benefit-risk of doing it yourself. In any case, as with many types of primary research, you can introduce self-reporting bias; where the people that respond do so because they are more likely to respond that others. This type of bias is most common in mass mailing of questionnaires which is, for many practices, the most common type of market research project.

Surveys

A survey is, quite simply, a technique to obtain the opinions of a group of people or members of a specific population. Surveys can be conducted in a number of ways, including using interviewing techniques as described above. Most often, surveys are conducted as either mailed-out instruments (questionnaires) or through phone calls, such as is common during election years to obtain opinion polls. In any type of survey, the questions are normally structured and standardized. Ideally, the questions are tested first with a sample of the population to be surveyed in order to ensure that the questions are interpreted as they are meant to be based on the question design. The two main types of surveys are researcher-administered, such as with interviews or phone calls. The other is self-administered, such as with patient satisfaction questionnaires or instruments that are sent to individuals via mail or e-mail.

Pros. One of the advantages to survey-type studies is that they can be conducted quickly and can encompass large samples with a single mailing or call program. As a result, when calculating reach per 1000 population, surveys are initially seen as quite cost effective. In a mailing, the primary expense is the cost of the mailing list and stamps, if sent via postal service. Consider that the majority of these types of projects are anonymous for the respondent (at least the respondent thinks they are); therefore, those that are typically shy, subject to the influence of group dynamics, or uncomfortable revealing personal information about themselves might be more likely to respond. There is also the advantage of eliminating interviewer bias, which is not uncommon in interviews, focus groups, and opinion polls.

Cons. The biggest downside of a mass survey is the GIGO effect: a single bad or poorly worded question will result in a loss of the value of all of the responses, which could be key for interpreting other areas of the study. It is often recommended that, even in these types of auto-controlled studies, an expert is involved in the survey design. Another risk is low response rate, which, of itself, can negate the value of this type of study. If, for example, you send out 10,000 surveys and get only 100 back, the statistical value of the study may be so small that any decisions made based on the results would pose a greater risk to the project. Along with this is the problem of self reporting bias; respondents represent some extreme portion of the population, such as those with an axe to grind or those with a particularly strong opinion about the issues being discussed. This results in the potential for skewed results and, subsequently, poor strategic decision making. Other problems involve the loss of control of the respondent, such as those that skip questions or who need clarification on a question but don't have anyone but a friend to ask.

Personal Observation

Personal observation differs from interviews and focus groups in that no questions are asked, no discussion is involved, and the observation is most times anonymous such that the person or persons being observed have no idea it is taking place.

Pros. The main advantage of personal observation is just that—personal observation. And the fact that it occurs in the actual environment in which a situation actually occurs is a huge benefit over methods such as simulation or envisioning. For example, if you want to know why patients report a longer wait time than is recorded (in the waiting room), you can set up cameras or a two-way mirror and study facial expressions, body language, and interactions. You may find, for example, that some seats place people in proximity to others that is too close for comfort, and, as a result, those chairs remain empty while patients resort to standing rather than sitting. This is also a good technique for studying the communication between the doctor and the patient in the exam room—very often a determinant as to whether an error or injury will result in a mal-practice lawsuit. These advantages allow for a much greater control of the study in that you can observe who you want when you want, which is often a critical component of the results being sought.

Cons. The first and most important risk of personal observation is the risk of compromising privacy. For example, having cameras anywhere in a medical practice may violate HIPAA privacy standards and laws, and, therefore, competent legal counsel should be consulted prior to initiation of this type of study. Even the mere act of observing a patient-physician interaction in an exam room without the patient's knowledge (which is the key to this method) may violate privacy laws and standards. In addition, it may be intrusive in that there is a loss of anonymity; the person knows he or she is being observed, such as through personal presence of the observer or obviated through the placement of cameras. The fact is, when individuals know they are being observed, they will often change their behavior; and then, the only benefit is to observe how a person acts when, well, he or she is being observed. Finally (and this may be painfully obvious), you need to have someone to observe. It requires, in the greatest sense, customers. If the practice is small or has few patients (or staff members, if observing them is the purpose of the study), it may affect the validity of the study results.

Customer Complaints

Similar to some of the other methods discussed here, this particular model is focused only on the negative reactions that customers have toward the practice. These may include patients, staff, payers, the general public, etc. The goal here is to intercept potential problems while they are localized and address them before they become systemic. This requires a greater resolve on the part of the researchers, particularly if they are employees of the practice, as not everyone is able to handle criticism (deserved or undeserved) well.

Pros. By examining customer complaints, you get a first-hand look at those things that interfere with the potential success of the practice from a first-level look. For example, if you replaced the front-office staff and you begin getting complaints about phone handling, you may want to make some calls yourself to uncover the cause of a potential problem. Or if staff members begin complaining about a particular issue, such as a new department head, supervisor, provider, or even environmental issues, this allows you to address it immediately before it grows into a crisis. Any method that adds specificity to a study allows an easier and more effective method to categorize data. In the case of complaints, it may allow you to create a set of buckets that can be used to organize complaints, such as waiting time, provider issues, staff problems, etc. In this way, you can also quantify complaints and develop policies for addressing them when a certain level or ratio is met.

Cons. One problem with this method has to do with self-reporting bias. For example, many people who are unhappy with a situation will not complain for a number of different reasons. On the other hand, when people do complain, their complaints are often emotionally driven and overstated. In many cases, the threshold for a complaint can be so high that by the time you hear about it, a crisis is already looming.

KANO MODEL

The Kano model actually falls under VOC and is a natural outcome of VOC work, such as discussed above. The purpose of the Kano model is to base attributes of products and services as they are perceived by the customer (patient, payer, staff, etc.). The Kano model is used to differentiate between what the customer wants and what the customer needs. For example, when traveling by air, a customer "need" may be as simple as walking off the airplane without injury. A "want" may be leaving or arriving on time, being treated courteously by the staff, or being offered snacks and drinks. In addition, the Kano model describes what are called "delighters," or consumer experiences that are unexpected and pleasurable. For example, being upgraded from coach to first class would be a delighter.

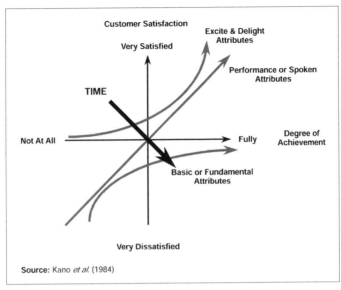

FIGURE 16. Kano model.

Attributes

In some of the literature, the formal components are known as threshold, performance, and excitement, which equate to basic needs, wants, and delighters, as described above and illustrated in Figure 16.

Threshold Attributes

The lowest of the Kano attributes is known as a threshold attribute, or, alternately, a basic attribute. These equate to basic or essential needs a customer has regarding the specific product or service being offered. In healthcare, this would be a proper diagnosis or treatment. Regarding a surgical procedure, a threshold attribute would be defined as a successful event; whether a successful outcome from the surgery, or, to some patients, just waking up after the event. Interestingly enough, increasing performance of threshold attributes results in diminishing returns since, by definition, these are as basic as can be attained.

It is difficult, for example, to improve on the proper diagnosis and treatment unless, of course, quality is an issue in the practice. And defining a surgical procedure as successful or not is also quite basic considering that success has been defined in advance by the patient and/or the provider. Improving on these, when the basic level of accomplishment is so fixed, requires huge resources and results in minimal benefit. On the other hand, failure to provide this level of attribute ultimately results in the failure of the product or service. Improper diagnosis and treatment creates a failure of the encounter. In air travel, for example, the threshold attribute for me is to walk away from a landing under my own power. If this doesn't happen, then the entire travel event is a failure.

Performance Attributes

Assuming that the threshold attributes are met and the product or service lives on, the next level entails the performance attributes, or those things that equate to a customer's requirements, or wants. These are events or tasks that add to the experience, such as not waiting too long to see the provider or being treated courteously and professionally by the staff. Considering my travel example, this would include arriving at the right airport on time. Contrary to the threshold attribute, here, more is normally considered better. Better treatment, shorter wait times, more perks, etc. will almost always equate to higher customer satisfaction levels.

Often, these performance attributes can be used to estimate what a customer is willing to pay.

As the level of these increases, so will the ability to charge more for the same basic service. This is one key to the success of many concierge healthcare programs that have begun to spring up around the country in the past few years. And it's not just what the customers are willing to pay; it also equates to just how much they are willing to tolerate before jumping ship and finding another provider. When assessing customer satisfaction including performance attributes, 10-point Likert scales are quite effective as they give the respondents a bit more freedom in expressing their opinions.

Excitement Attributes

Excitement attributes are often times called delighters, and unlike performance attributes, are mostly unexpected. For example, receiving a phone call from the provider the evening of the visit to check on the patient is very often noted by patients as the number one exciter related to a visit. Some practices offer wireless Internet to allow patients to work or play in the waiting room. Faxing or e-mailing patients their test results with a short comment or interpretation (without them having to beg and plead to get these) is a real exciter for many patients. Again, from a travel perspective, this might include being upgraded from coach to first class on a long flight.

Like performance attributes, presence of excitement attributes can significantly increase patient satisfaction, although it takes far less mass in this area to accomplish the same results. Unlike performance attributes, absence of these will normally not result in a reduction in patient satisfaction because, as stated above, they are mostly not expected. Excitement attributes will often tip the competitive balance for a business, particularly when there are larger sums of money involved. All things being equal (referring to quality of care and outcomes), an employer with very happy employees may offer a practice a "preferred" status, increasing referrals, or a payer may negotiate better rates based on higher patient satisfaction ratings (yes, it does happen). In many cases, direct referrals can be positively affected through the offering of this type of attribute.

Frustraters

Frustraters are not necessarily an official part of the Kano model; however, they are often key components relating to customer satisfaction. In fact, a frustrater can undo many of the benefits found in the last two attributes. This attribute creates wait time, confusion, and frustration for a customer. Some examples are the inability to navigate the phone system and talk to a live person, or not being able to get the practice to respond with lab results when promised. Many times, frustraters are the result of poor communication created by either the staff or the patient, or in some cases, both. The presence of a single frustrater, such as excessive wait time to see the provider, can negate or degrade an otherwise positive patient experience. Frustraters will almost always have a negative impact on satisfaction surveys, and people who are victims of this attribute may often make it their job to tell everyone they know about their negative experience.

Alternate Kano Designs

In addition to the graph shown in Figure 16, a Kano model can be represented as a table that lists the attributes necessary for the patient to have a positive experience (Figure 17).

The key is to know how to define these from the patients' perspective, and the only way to do this is to ask. The only way you can build a practice that is customer-focused is to involve the customer in the visit experience. This includes patients as well as payers, staff, employers, and everyone else defined as your customer. You may think you know what they want but too often that assumption results in the need to rework your model— waste that can be avoided with proper planning.

Overall, the Kano model is a powerful tool for shaping what you are going to offer in the future. It provides the practice with the ability to understand from marketing and sales what it needs to communicate to the marketplace in order to bring in additional business. The bottom line is this: to have a successful practice, you need to focus on the customer,

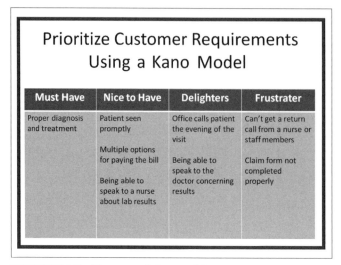

FIGURE 17. **Kano model as a table.**

and this tool allows you to formalize that process, create a measurement system for your efforts, and analyze the results of your work flow, and it provides a perfect avenue for continuous process improvement.

CRITICAL TO QUALITY

Critical to Quality (CTQ) is a tool that follows VOC and Kano model in natural sequence. VOC, through the use of interview and survey techniques, has helped you to link up with your customers to identify what it is they want and expect from you as a medical practice. The Kano model helped to organize this information into a qualitative model used to better define what it is the customer is saying. Now, it is time to create a set of metrics that will enable you to begin quantifying your current state as it applies to this information and help design a future state that is oriented to your customers—whether patients, family, payers, employers, or staff.

The CTQ tree is sometimes called an affinity diagram, and it is an ordered, graphical representation of the drivers behind the attributes defined in the Kano model. For example, the customer "needs" a proper diagnosis and treatment, and the CTQ defines the drivers that are required for that to happen. Then, it takes those drivers, which are, for the most part, qualitative, and helps to define the metrics that will be used to measure your relative level of success or failure. These might include how well the treatment worked measured in outcomes or as a follow-up, as a percent of the time that the diagnosis was correct vs. the times it had to be modified. Using CTQ, you create a process map of sorts, referred to

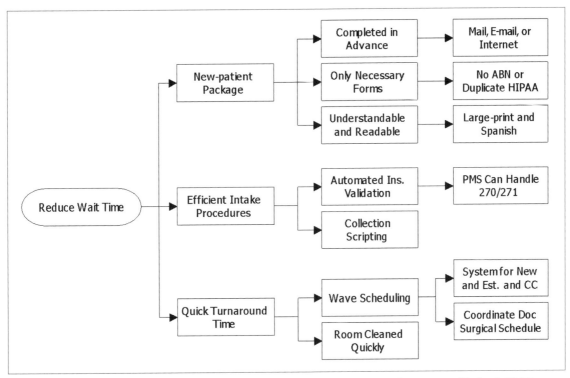

FIGURE 18. **CTQ tree. ABN, Advance Beneficiary Notice; CC, consult; Est, established; PMS, practice management system.**

as a CTQ tree, that increases the granularity of the qualitative components until such time as you reach a level that requires metrics.

Critical-to-Quality Tree

A CTQ tree, as described above, is a graphical representation of the drivers behind VOC and Kano attributes. While not a rule, we often find that the tree extends to four levels, including the initial reference. In any case, the tree stops when you get to the point where the next driver requires specific metrics, such as wait time or travel distance, etc. These will be handled as part of the key performance indicator (KPI) matrix, introduced later. The tree begins with a single qualitative reference, such as wait time, treatment modality, transportation efficiency, or any other customer complaint, satisfaction, or concern. The second level identifies the main drivers for that reference. In Figure 18, we list wait time as a key qualitative issue for patients.

The three most critical drivers that affect wait time are the new patient package, intake procedures, and room turnaround times. The third level lists the drivers that affect the second level drivers. In our example, we find that what types of forms and the ability for the patient to read and understand them are key drivers behind the new patient package, particularly if our goal is to optimize efficiency and minimize completion time. To effect quick turnaround time, the key drivers would be the manner in which patients are scheduled and how quickly the room can be cleaned between patients. In some cases, you might stop here, particularly if the next step involved measurements, such as with the Room Cleaned Quickly driver. Here, the next logical step would be developing a metric and measurement system to see just how long it takes to get a room turned around between patients. Otherwise, you go to level four, which, as before, defines the related drivers in the previous level.

In our example, we might find that in order to effect more efficient scheduling, we need a system that can differentiate visit times for new and established patients, and it requires that we coordinate surgical schedules so we don't have patients scheduled with a provider that is in a scheduled surgery at the same time. Note that, in our example, the next logical step for the majority of drivers is to begin developing metrics for each of our drivers. For example, under the second level of Efficient Intake Procedures, our final driver is to determine whether the system can handle 270/271 forms for automated insurance verification. Here, we might develop a metric that is a pass/fail measurement of the times that this worked vs. the times that it didn't. We might also continue to a denial analysis and measure how often the claim was denied due to insurance verification as a percentage of all 270s submitted.

Key Performance Indicators

KPIs are quantifiable measurements, agreed to beforehand, that reflect the critical success factors of an organization. A medical practice may have as a KPI the time it takes from a patient call (or a referral) to appointment or the time a patient spends in the waiting room. Using instruments like SF-12 and SF-36, a practice may have as a KPI the outcomes in terms of quality of life for a patient after a procedure or a series of treatments. Perhaps the practice has decided that all phone calls will be answered within 15 seconds, and alternately, missed calls will be returned within one hour. Whatever KPIs are decided upon, they should reflect the practice's goals and be key to its success (as defined by the stakeholders), and they must be quantifiable (measurable). If the practice is looking to incorporate these for the long haul, it is important that the measurement systems established remain consistent. Figure 19 is an example of a KPI diagram.

For example, if measuring wait time, start and stop events need to be identified. Does the clock start when the patient arrives or at the time the appointment was scheduled (deals

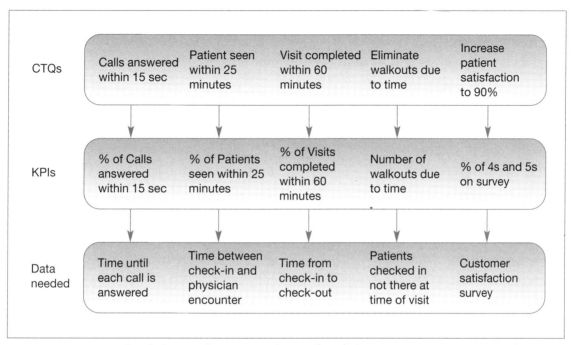

FIGURE 19. Example of a key performance indicator (KPI) diagram. CTQ, critical to quality.

with later and/or early patients)? Does the clock start when the phone starts its ring or after the first ring (a ring tone can last as long as 3 seconds, and if 15 seconds is the goal, that can account for fully 20% of the measured time)? To construct a KPI diagram, three things are required: the CTQ as defined in the diagram (or tree); the KPI itself; and a description of the actual data needed.

In our example here, we have defined being able to answer the phone within 15 seconds as CTQ for our practice. In order to accomplish this, the KPI would be the percent of calls answered within that 15-second time period. The data we would need would be the actual time from our defined start until the phone was answered. It may seem simple or, to many, common sense, but without a structured, defined, and documented approach, we often find that we drift from our original intentions or in many cases, staff turnover creates new ideas on how metrics should be collected or measurements made.

Note that KPIs are not just limited to patient issues. They are also used to improve and track business and compliance issues, such as accounts receivable (A/R), denial rates, E/M compliance, etc. For example, if my CTQ is a denial rate below 5%, my KPI might be the number of denials as a percent of all claim lines submitted, and the data needed would be total denials and total claim lines submitted. If another CTQ (from a business perspective) was to have my A/R under 45 days, my KPI might be average A/R, either total or for specific (or all) payers. The data needed would be time from date of service (or submission date) to final posting of that claim. I might want to collect these data by payer or even patient type or specialty. Remember, without CTQ, you don't have a customer-driven business and without that, particularly in an industry like healthcare, you won't have your practice for very long.

SIPOC

SIPOC, an acronym for Suppliers, Inputs, Process Steps, Outputs, and Customers, is used as a high-level tool to define the overall operation of a particular process; procedure; or, at the highest level, the organization as a whole. Many practices find the SIPOC tool difficult to use due to the need to define both suppliers and customers. In industry, a supplier is one who "supplies" the business with the products it needs in order to function. In manufacturing, this might be the company that supplies raw materials. In retail, it would be a supplier of finished products. In the airline industry, it would define the entity that supplies fliers, such as Orbitz, Travelocity, travel agencies, or even the airlines' own Web sites.

In a medical practice, the supplier is the entity that supplies the patient. This could be the payer (provider member directory), the patient or patient family, another physician (as a referral), or even the employer who self-insures the patient. The customer is often the same person and, again, that creates a bit of confusion for many medical practices. The customer, as defined earlier, can be the person who receives the product or service, pays for the product or service, or benefits from the product or service. Directly, we consider the patient as our primary customer. In many cases, it is the family that supervises a visit or encounter. The payer ultimately pays for the service, and the employer (hopefully) benefits from the encounter by taking care of its employees. Inputs represent all of the data that are necessarily collected in order for the process to work and might include intake forms; medical history and exam results; the superbill or encounter form; and, from a process improvement perspective, measurements of time within the visit cycle itself. The process map is a high-level look at the process itself, noting only the primary steps involved. Outputs represent the data that are collected as a result of the process (in our example, a patient visit) and might include the treatment plan; a CMS-1500 form or 837 file; a patient care form if a procedure was performed; and, following with our process improvement example, the result of the time measurements from the visit cycle. Figure 20 shows an example of a SIPOC diagram for a patient visit.

SIPOC diagrams are, for the most part, the initial step for project selection and management and should be completed in every case.

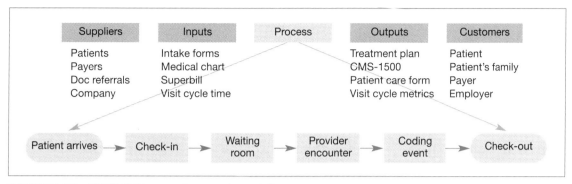

FIGURE 20. **SIPOC diagram for a patient visit.**

SPAGHETTI DIAGRAM

Let's start with a pretty official definition: A spaghetti diagram is a method that uses a continuous line to trace the path and distance traveled of a particular object or person throughout a process. It is most commonly illustrated on a floor map diagram that contains the entire process being evaluated, such as a hospital floor or medical office layout. The purpose of this tool is to help with identifying movements and layouts that create unnecessary movement and travel distance between steps in the process.

This tool has proven itself to be highly effective in evaluating transportation processes in hospitals, particularly for patients traveling to and from their rooms to the lab, radiology, or the operating room. In an office setting, it may seem less important since for many of us, the distances patients travel seem to be limited. In a hospital, patients are often wheeled around in chairs or on gurneys, while in our offices it is the feet that do the work. So why would travel distance be an issue? Let's look at some data.

Depending on the study you read, men in their thirties and forties walk comfortably somewhere between 6.5 and 7.5 feet per second (4.4 and 5.1 mph, respectively). In a small office, a patient may travel 70 feet from the door to the check-in counter and then to a seat in the waiting room. From the waiting room, let's say its 140 feet to get to the exam room. From the exam room back to the waiting area to check out is another 140 feet and then another 30 feet out the door. So, the entire distance traveled by the patient is 380 feet, including all travel. At an average rate of 7 feet per second, the travel portion of the visit would take approximately 54 seconds. Not bad, actually.

Now, let's move on a few years and see how much time it might take someone in their seventies. Comfortable walking speeds drop to around 5 feet per second for healthy people in their seventies. For one of these folks, the trip would take around 76 seconds, or 1 minute and 16 seconds; and remember, these are for healthy, active adults, not people who have health problems that, in some cases, can add minutes to a trip such as described above. It still may not seem like a lot of time but let's say we can shave 30 seconds off each patient visit by organizing the rooms more efficiently.

For example, let's say that, in our sample practice, 38% of patients show up for a specific treatment, such as an injection. If we knew this in advance (which, of course, we would by the appointment type), we could allocate a room close to the waiting room for these treatments since they consume a significant portion of the work effort in the practice. If the practice sees 70 patients a day, 30 seconds per patient translates to around 35 minutes per day, or around 150 hours per year. Realistically (this is an important point to avoid exaggerating the benefits of this tool), we are not going to be able to convert all of the time savings into dollars, but even if we could associate a 25% conversion, that's around 35 hours per year. If you can process a patient every 15 minutes (cycle time, not visit time), and you generate $80 per encounter, this would translate into $11,200 dollars per year; not easy to ignore. This exemplifies the purpose of Lean Six Sigma as a process improvement model—increasing profitability by improving efficiency. Seeing more patients or performing more procedures without any additional overhead adds 100% to the bottom line.

Another example involves location of the physicians' offices. In one practice for which I did a project similar to this, the practice was in the shape of a big square so that you could start at the waiting room door, walk around a large square, and end up back at the waiting room. Lab and treatment rooms were in the center, and patient rooms and offices were around the perimeter. In this case, the physicians' had their offices to the left and right of the waiting room door, and the exam rooms were along the back part of the square, the farthest point from the waiting room. On average, patients traveled 140 feet more than they needed to. From a mathematical point of view, when you average the high-steppers and the shufflers, it wasted around 31 seconds per patient. At 150 patients per day, this came out to around 336 wasted hours and 1034 unnecessary miles traveled each year. And we haven't even talked about the amount of wasted time that staff and physicians spend going to and fro in an inefficiently designed office. The bottom line is this: every minute a provider spends waiting for a patient subtracts revenue from the profit margin, and every wasted minute (and foot) patients spend getting seen and treated adds to their frustration and dissatisfaction.

How to Use the Spaghetti Diagram

When getting ready to spaghetti diagram a process, there are two points to remember. First, this is a continuous event; you go from beginning to end. The second point is similar to the

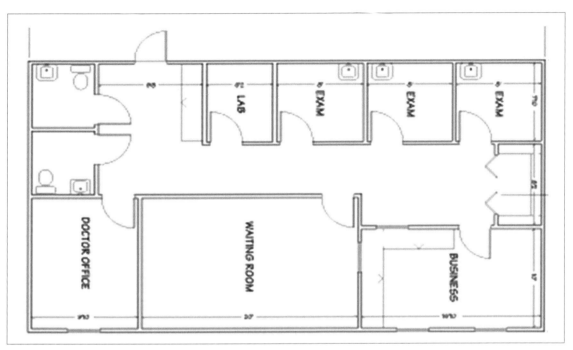

FIGURE 21. **Floor plan for a small medical practice.**

first in that this should represent the entire trip a patient (or staff member or physician or lab specimen) travels during the event (encounter, procedure, meeting, etc.), hence the idea that once the tip of the writing device hits the paper, it stays there until the event is over.

Start by printing (or projecting onto a white board) the physical layout of the building, facility, or similar type of structure where the event takes place. Floor plans work well as do blueprints, as long as there isn't too much detail beyond the basic layout of the rooms, hallways, offices, etc. (Figure 21).

The first step in creating the diagram is to identify the object you wish to track (claim form, person, piece of equipment, etc.) and its starting point on the diagram. For example, if tracking a patient for a visit, you could start at the check-in desk or the front door; or, if trying to evaluate the entire distance traveled, even in the parking lot that leads into the office. Then move the pen or pencil around the floor plan to approximately replicate the movement the object takes. Keep the pen to the paper until the entire travel event is terminated. A common mistake that people make is to draw the line through walls or to not trace the stairs, but to do this does not give a realistic representation of the actual flow.

If you do this correctly, you will begin to notice that the line begins to look like a line of spaghetti; hence its name. When complete, you should be able to estimate the approximate distance the object traveled for this event. From a strategic standpoint, the purpose

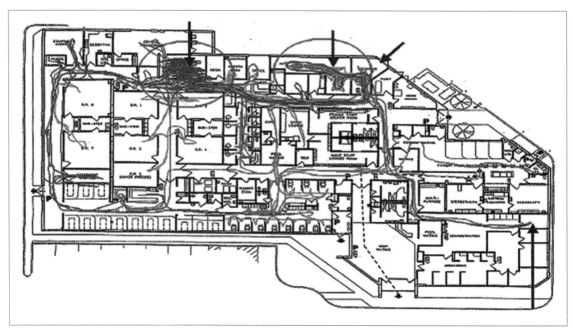

FIGURE 22. **Spaghetti diagram of a surgical center.**

of this tool is to identify, from the diagram and the layout, which parts of the travel event are not necessary, could be shortened, or could be consolidated, or other actions that could be taken to shorten the time and distance required.

Figure 22 is an example of a spaghetti diagram of a surgical center. Each of the different lines represents a different object, such as a patient, a staff member, or even materials that are moved around for surgical access.

Figure 23 is an example of a large medical clinic, showing the travel route of a series of typical patient visits. It includes not only the patient movement, but the movement of the staff, providers, and other clinical personnel in support of the visit event. In this case, the number of trips to the nursing station, supply room, kitchen, and other areas were counted to see if there was a way to reduce the amount of waste and redundancy discovered.

DATA MINING AND STATISTICS

Often treated as interchangeable, data mining and statistical analyses are two distinctly different, yet related, areas. Data mining is the exploration of an analysis of a large amount of data in order to discover valid, novel, and understandable patterns in the data. Statistics, on the other hand, is a mathematical science that is defined by the collection, analysis, interpretation, and presentation of data. Data mining and statistics are listed here as a single

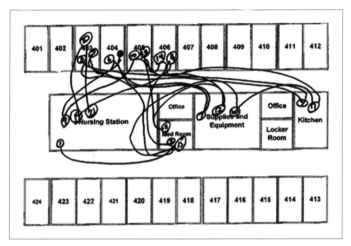

FIGURE 23. Spaghetti diagram of a large medical clinic.

tool in that, for the purposes of our discussion, they are both used in the processes of discovery, correlation, and cause and effect. Some might argue that they are not tools at all, but rather an entire area of process improvement. And I would be one to agree, except that to do justice to this as more than a tool would require a separate book. In fact, there are hundreds if not thousands of books written on the topics of data mining and statistics, and it would behoove the reader to continue on his or her own to study these areas of process improvement.

In nearly every industry, middle to upper management have a strong, if not a perfunctory understanding of business statistics, and this should also be true for medical practices. When challenged under a Recovery Audit Contractor (RAC) audit, we should be able to determine if the sample was random, if the sample size is statistically valid, and if the populations being studied are similar, and be able to conduct tests to determine whether the audit results are significant or, as I have often found, just full of hot air. The same is true when looking at costs or collections or conducting a provider performance analysis. How about when considering whether to accept a contract from a payer? Data mining and statistics are powerful tools for assessing the value and overall profitability of a contract. Just as these tools are used in the furtherance of clinical quality, so they should also be used in the furtherance of business profitability.

Data Mining vs. Statistics

Data mining was originally developed to act as an expert system to solve problems. It is less interested in the mechanics of the technique and more interested in the results. A common thread with data mining is if it makes sense, we use it. Although we are careful to validate the source of the data, it doesn't require any assumptions to be made, such as distribution. Data mining is more about pattern recognition and discovery and is very helpful in finding patterns in very large amounts of data.

For example, data mining is a great way to discover potential problems related to wait time, A/R issues, or claims processing delays. While it doesn't require a deep understanding of math, it does require that the person conducting the study have a decent understanding of data and data organization as well as the business problem being studied.

Statistics, on the other hand, consists of a set of tests that measure the correctness of the data models being used. It begs the question about whether the assumptions of the data or the models are correct. For example, is the R^2 (correlation of coefficient) high enough to explain the meaning of a relationship? Statistics also involves hypothesis testing, which can be used to measure the significance of a relationship between two data or more sets of data. In this case, unlike data mining, statistics is sensitive to the distribution of the data; particularly whether it is normally or non-normally distributed. Whereas data mining looks at an entire database, statistics tends to rely more on sampling—both size and technique. And unlike studying large databases for patterns, statistical analyses usually requires the analyst to not only have a good background in the data and the business problem, but also strong statistical skills. Remember, data mining depends on size while statistics depends on criticality.

What Types of Data Do You Want?

The types of data you need (or want) are dependent on the types of studies you want to conduct or the processes you want to examine. If looking at A/R issues, you would want to see historical data for billing and collections—date of service vs. submission vs. posting dates. You might conduct a study of the billing cycle time to see if there are bottlenecks creating increases in average A/R days. If you are conducting a fee analysis, you would certainly need your current fee schedule and maybe the number of times that each procedure code/modifier group was billed out. Maybe an examination of payer mix would be in order as would be a review of the average charges for other physicians in your specialty across your state and possibly the nation. For a provider performance analysis, you would need a database that related the number of times each provider reported each procedure code/modifier group and even a retrospective denial audit to see whether what was billed related to what was paid. You might also need external comparative data sets, such as the RVS Update Committee (RUC) time study and the RBRVS or physician fee schedule database. Concerning

VOC, you would want to see the results of patient satisfaction studies or even look at complaint data, including time-to-resolution.

What Kind of Statistics Do You Want?

For some of us, determining the kind and type of statistics we need is easier than for others: NONE. But the truth is, without the use of statistics, you might never go beyond the step of discovery and might never have the ability to defend yourself against external audits, reviews, and other payer and government attacks. And remember, what follows is in no way a substitution for a good class or introductory book on statistics. What follows is only a set of references to the types of statistical tests and techniques that are very valuable for the practice.

Distribution Families. One of the most important areas of statistics is actually probability; at least with regard to defining the distribution family represented by the data. We are all used to seeing what is referred to as the "bell curve," because it looks like a bell. This is also called the normal distribution curve and is an entire statistical model within itself. Normally distributed data follow a specific set of rules that make it relatively simple to understand and estimate the nature of our data. Too often, however, people don't understand distributions or just assume that all data are normally distributed, and this leads only to making bad business decisions on bad data. Distributions can be separated by the types of variables, such as discrete or continuous. Some distributions are useful for predicting staffing activity, such as the Poisson distribution, which follow a pattern of counting, such as how many phone calls to expect per hour or even at a specific hour of the day.

Measures of Central Tendency. The most common and useful of statistical measurements are measurements of central tendency, primarily the mean, the median, and the mode. The mean (commonly known as the arithmetic average, or just average), represents the center of a set of values and is highly sensitive to outliers, or individual values that are significantly higher or lower than the majority of the values in the database. This is quite often true with conversion factor (CF) calculations, where you might find the majority to be somewhere between 60 and 100, but then there are some that have values in excess of 600 or 700. The mean also does not always consider the frequency with which values are reported and, as such, gives each value an equal share of the sample. For example, if you were to try to calculate the average CF from a fee schedule, you would miss the significance of the frequency by which the procedures were reported. If you have two procedures, one performed 1000 times and one performed 10 times, a typical situation would give each of the individual CF amounts an equal say in calculating the average. When the data are normally distributed (or approximately normally distributed) or you have a large sample (say, in excess of 100 data points), the mean can be a very robust and valuable measurement.

The location of the median, on the other hand, is positional. Instead of measuring the central point of the sum of the values for each data point, it measures the central location of the set of data points. For example, if you have 100 data points, to calculate the mean, you would add them all up and divide by 100. To calculate the median, you would list them on a spreadsheet in ascending order and pick the middle value (in this case, the average of the values at positions 50 and 51). The median is much less susceptible to outliers and therefore is a better choice for data that may not be normally distributed, such as CF values or times.

The mode is a measurement of the frequency for which a value is reported. For example, if you reported procedure X 25 times, procedure Y 23 times, and procedure Z 58 times, the mode would be 58. This is not as robust a measure of central tendency as it is a measure of event activity.

Measures of Variability. Knowing where the center resides in a set of data points is very important but understanding the variability is just as important. Variability is a measurement of the average distance, if you will, that the individual data points within a database differ from the actual central measurement. For example, let's say you have a set of data representing the first nine months of collection percentages for each of two physicians, as follows:

- **Doctor 1**
  - January   26%
  - February   28%
  - March   49%
  - April   38%
  - May   45%
  - June   51%
  - July   74%
  - August   38%
  - September 47%
- **Doctor 2**
  - January   44%
  - February   34%

— March   50%
— April   44%
— May   38%
— June   37%
— July   51%
— August   45%
— September 53%

Both sets of collection data have an average of 44%, yet for Doctor 1, the collection percent values range from a low of 26% to a high of 74%, while the collection percent values for Doctor 2 range from a low of 34% to a high of 53%. Here, it is quite clear that, even though both have the same average collection amount during the same period, Doctor 2 showed a much higher degree of consistency from month to month. In effect, the variation of the collection percent for Doctor 2 was considerably lower than for Doctor 1.

When looking at variability for values with normal distributions, we tend to use the standard deviation, which is the average of the squared differences between each data point and the average within a given data set. For non-normally distributed data, we tend to use what is called the interquartile ratio (IQR), or the difference between the 25th percentile (the middle of the lower half) and the 75th percentile (the middle of the upper half) of any given set of data.

Sample Error.   One of the key ideas behind inferential statistics is being able to estimate the degree of accuracy that is present within any sampling of a population. For example, if we look at the nine months of collection data for Doctor 1 in the example above, we have calculated the average collection as 44%. But is it really 44%? And if this doctor reported a collection amount next month of 40%, what would be the significance, if any, of that 4% difference? Confidence intervals allow us to calculate the expected range of significance for any set of values based on two parameters: the standard deviation (variability) and the size of the sample. The greater the size, the greater our confidence in the results and, subsequently, the smaller the confidence interval. The smaller the variability, the greater our confidence in the results and hence, once again, the smaller the confidence interval.

In our example here, we are only addressing the statistic of a confidence interval around a mean. There are other types of confidence intervals, such as around a median or dealing with proportions rather than these types of values. In our example, the average is 44% but the 95% confidence interval is between 33% and 55%. This means that we can be 95% confident that, if we were to pull another sample of nine months of collections from this provider (all else being equal), the average collection amount for that period would be between 33% and 55%. This also allows us to assign significance to a mean, such that we can recognize that the differences between the mean and that lower and upper bounds are due to normal variability, or noise. Notice that with Doctor 2, while we still have a mean of 44%, the 95% confidence interval is between 39% and 49%; a much smaller range due to a smaller measure of variability (standard deviation of 6.6 vs. 14.3 for Doctor 1).

Correlation and Regression.   Correlation is a mathematical measurement of the strength and direction of the relationship between two variables represented in a database. For example, you might want to know if patient satisfaction scores are related to wait times or if no-shows have any relation (and if so, how strong and in what direction) to the length of time it takes from making an appointment to getting to see the doctor. Maybe you want to know if there is a relationship between payer mix and A/R or denial rates and billing systems.

Correlation is a powerful tool and uses a single value, known as a Pearson's-r (from now on, we will just call it r), to measure the correlation of the variables. The value of r can range from -1 to $+1$. The sign indicates the direction of the relationship. For example, shorter people tend to weigh less, so if you associated weight to height, you would see a pretty good positive correlation. On the other hand, the less a car weighs, the better the gas mileage, and so here, you would see a negative r value. The strength of the relationship is also measured by r, with -1 being a perfect inverse relationship and $+1$ being a perfect linear relationship (linearity is very important but left for another day). An r value of 0 would indicate that the data are completely random with respect to the two variables, and there isn't any relationship at all.

Regression goes hand in hand with correlation and is used to calculate the slope of the line that best fits the relationship of the two variables being measured. For example, I plot two variables on a graph; x equals the amount I charge for each procedure, and y equals the RVU for that same procedure. I am looking to see if my fees are related to the Medicare fee schedule. The graph indicates that they are, in fact, related with an r value of $+.8$; pretty high on a scale of 0 to 1. Using regression, we would draw a line through the points on the scatter graph that would indicate the slope of that relationship, which further allows us to make predictions about the relationship (or actual value) of a variable compared to another with the range of our data. The slope line is calculated to be what is known as the "best fit" line, meaning that it best represents the average relationship of the variables throughout the length of the database. Most often, this is done using something called "least means squared," and simply put (I think), just means that the line is drawn such that the distance between the point on the line and the actual point where the two variables intersect is the least value possible.

Hypothesis Testing. The last (sort of) statistic that is used quite often in process improvement projects is hypothesis testing. Quite often, we want to see if there is a significant difference between a set of values or one proportion compared to a population or the means of two sets of data, etc. To do this, we employ hypothesis testing. For example, let's say that you analyze another nine months of data for Doctor 2 and come up with an average collection for those nine months of 36%. You want to know if that is significantly different from the 44% average that you calculated prior. To do this, you could conduct a hypothesis test where you compare the average of 44% based on the nine months of data against the 36% average value. In this case, you find that the 36% is significantly different and could use this to move forward in determining why the difference occurred.

In hypothesis testing, the basic concept is innocent unless proven guilty. In essence, you start with the assumption that there isn't any difference between the variables or the data (null hypothesis) and then test to see if you are wrong. Hypothesis testing involves establishing certain parameters that are, unfortunately, way beyond the scope of this book. Things like beta (the risk you are willing to take of saying there isn't a difference when there is), alpha (the risk of saying there is a difference when there isn't), power (which is 1-beta), the probability of an exception occurring by random chance (p-value), and other fun stuff like that.

The bottom line is, this is not the time or the place to teach a basic course in statistics but it is critical that at least the champions on a process improvement project have a basic understanding of this science. Books like *Statistics for Dummies* are a great primer. Or go to www.statistics.com and take a few introduction to statistics online courses. If you do, your eyes will be opened to a myriad of opportunities not only for process improvement but as an opportunity to protect your practice from poorly conducted audits and reviews and unscrupulous payer behavior.

ISHIKAWA DIAGRAM

Also known as "fishbone" or "cause-and-effect diagrams," the Ishikawa is the brainchild of Kaoru Ishikawa, a process- and quality-improvement engineer who worked for Kawasaki shipyards. The Ishikawa diagram is the first tool in a set of steps that focus on the topic of cause and effect.

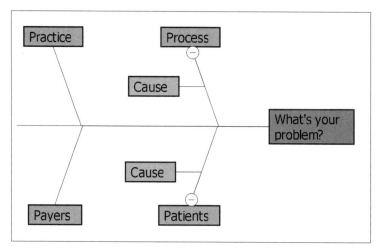

FIGURE 24. Ishikawa diagram.

The purpose of the fishbone diagram is to assist process improvement teams (or individuals) to categorize the often-times many different suspected causes of a specific problem or issue. It is very beneficial for structuring brainstorming sessions as it gives participants a visual representation of the vastness of the solutions available for a single focused problem. Pretty incredible, actually! So often, during problem-solving sessions, we see suggestions as drift because they fall outside of a predetermined target zone. The beauty of the Ishikawa technique is that *every* suggestion, at least initially, is within that zone. It's only later, after a more intensive vetting process during which each potential solution is further assessed, that specific suggestions may fall off the target.

As seen in the Figure 24, the reason it is called a *fishbone diagram* is, well, the resemblance to a filleted fish. The problem statement is at the head, or right side of the diagram and each of the major categories that are used to group, or compartmentalize and all of the suggested causes for the problem statement are arranged around the "bones" that protrude from the spine

How to Develop a Fishbone Diagram

The first step in developing a fishbone diagram is to agree on a problem statement (effect). Write this down at the right side of the flip chart, paper, or white board; draw a box around it; and draw a horizontal arrow running to it from the left. This is the "backbone" of the diagram. Then, either through a simple selection process or, sometimes, brainstorming, select the major categories for causes of the problem. Here are some generic headings that are used quite often:

- Policies
- Payers
- People
- Patients
- Equipment
- Measurement
- Environment
- Technology

For each possible category of cause, extend a branch from the backbone, and list the category at the top (or the bottom). You can have as many or as few categories as necessary to address all issues. When the diagram is set, begin a brainstorming session on **all** possible causes of the problem. The word *all* is the operative word here. Remember, during brainstorming, no limits or filters are placed on suggestions (except for "no feedback to another suggestion"). The purpose is to encourage open and free movement around the table.

Sometimes, you may find that a suggestion fits into more than one category, such as insurance validation. This can be due to an old insurance card (re: patient), lack of an automated verification system (re: technology), bad information from the payer (re: payer), or even a lack of verification at all (re: policy). When this happens, list the cause under all applicable categories. Later, when you begin the vetting process, you will narrow these down to the most significant causes. The other thing that happens sometimes is that one suggestion is actually a subset of another suggestion. For example, one cause of excessive wait time may be due to poor scheduling (re: technology). Another cause suggested may be failure to get enough information on chief complaint prior to appointment, which could fall under the scheduling cause. In these cases, draw a branch (or another bone) from an existing cause and show it as a subset of that primary cause. When complete, your diagram might look something like the one shown in Figure 25.

As mentioned above, some diagrams will have several branches while others may have only one. Don't get hung up on symmetry by trying to force additional categories if they truly don't exist. Figure 26 is an example of a two-branch Ishikawa diagram created to better understand the cause of premature births at a medical center.

Once the brainstorming session has exhausted all possible suggestions (meaning that, in a team setting, everyone has passed), begin to review each of the suggestions from a high-level of criticality. The idea here is to go back, take some time to consider each of the suggestions, and eliminate those that are duplicates and/or may be applicable to the problem statement.

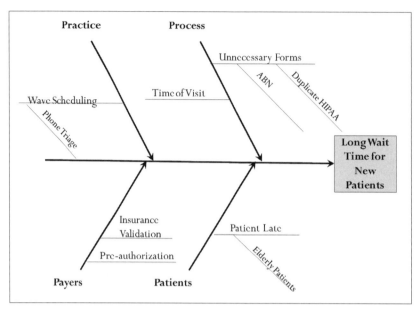

FIGURE 25. More complex Ishikawa diagram.

Sometimes, suggestions may require additional research or study to determine their validity. For example, someone may suggest that the PMS is not capable of producing certain reports or performing a given task. It would be important to make sure this is true before moving forward with the possibility of an improvement project. In this case, you might want to assign someone to contact support to verify whether the procedure or task can be accomplished. Interestingly, if it is and you didn't know about it, you could transfer the cause from, say, "technology" over to "people" and use it as an opportunity to arrange training for the staff. When the list has been whittled down to the "real" causes, begin a process of prioritization for testing and improvement. Be sure to focus on those causes that are most relevant and have the greatest benefit-to-risk ratio.

TAKT TIME

Now here is a bit of an arcane tool that initially didn't seem to have any kind of applicability within the medical practice. But with a bit of research, testing, and (if you will) retooling, it turns out that it does, indeed, have some applications that are quite important for benchmarking and estimating FTE requirements for a practice.

This tool is derived from the German word *taktzeit*, which translates to "clock" cycle. Product flow is expected to fall within a pace that is less than or equal to the Takt time. In manufacturing, it is used to measure the rate that a completed product needs to be finished in or-

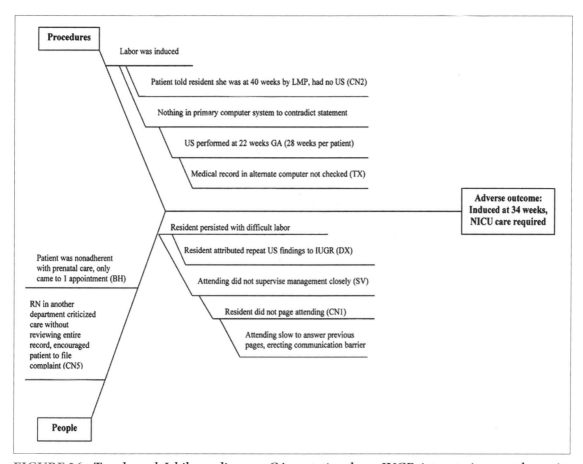

FIGURE 26. Two-branch Ishikawa diagram. GA, gestational age; IUGR, intrauterine growth restriction; LMP, last menstrual period; NICU, neonatal intensive care unit; US, ultrasound.

der to meet customer demand. If you have a Takt time of two minutes, that means every two minutes a complete product, assembly, or machine is produced off the line. In a medical practice, it is used to identify the required rate at which a patient needs to be processed or a test needs to be completed in order to meet expected volume or demand rate.

Takt time is not determined by the practice; meaning that it is not a goal that is set *a priori,* but rather is the result of existing flow within the system. In reality, you can never achieve 100% efficiency as there are always events, or unplanned variability, that leak into the day. There is a saying that goes something like this: "You can plan the picnic but you can't plan the weather." Translated, this means that you can schedule your day with patient visits, tests, procedures, etc., but you can't control patient no-shows, staff absences, emergencies, or other things that can get in the way of a smooth operation. Sometimes, losing a payer contract will result in lower patient volume, and when this happens, Takt time could (and should) be adjusted. Therefore, Takt time can be defined as the maximum time allowed to process an encounter or complete a test or procedure in order to meet demand.

Takt time is calculated by dividing the total amount of allocated time during a work day, period, or shift by the DDR, or in our case, the number of encounters, tests, or procedures. For example, let's say you have a practice that is open from 9:00 AM until 5:00 PM. This is eight hours. Multiply this by 60 to get 480 minutes. Subtract 30 minutes for unpaid lunch, breaks, cleanup, etc., and you end up with 450 minutes of staffed time. Divide this by the number of patients seen per day (30 for our example), and you get Takt time. In our example, this comes out to one encounter every 12.5 minutes. This doesn't mean that you "see" a patient or perform a procedure every 12.5 minutes; it means rather that you are staffed to manage a flow that requires a patient or procedure to be introduced into the cycle every 12.5 minutes (actually produced every 12.5 minutes, but that doesn't sound very good when dealing with healthcare encounters). The quicker a process can be completed (reduced Takt time), the more efficient the system.

Translating Takt to FTE

One challenge that practices face is benchmarking the number of FTEs required to operate the practice or facility. Too many, and you compromise profit; too few, and you compromise quality. Many practices use external data in order to estimate the number of FTEs of staff as a ratio to the number of providers. The concept is fine, but without a better understanding of how the control group of practices used for comparison is managed, it often becomes a crap-shoot. For example, how many hours of work define one FTE provider in a practice? What if some of the practices included in the study operate only 32 hours a week while some operate at 70? I know; you are thinking, "averages, my man, averages." That is all well and good *if and only if* you can define the parameters that are used to estimate the average, including estimates of error; and I have yet to see an existing data set that meets these requirements.

So, where do we go? Well, using Takt time is an interesting (and fun) beginning. I can't say that it is spot on as I haven't conducted a formal study of the results. I can say, however, that at least anecdotally, it is a pretty decent starting point from a manager's perspective.

The formula is this: cycle time multiplied by DDR divided by staffed time per day equals FTE requirements. Let's take another example to illustrate this. Let's say we have a practice that sees 78 patients per day (on average). This is the definition of DDR, or the number of patients that need to be processed during the work day. Our example practice is open and staffed (providing services) 10 hours per day (28,800 available seconds). The average cycle time for a patient visit (from check in to check out) is 72 minutes (4320 seconds). The formula would be as follows: [4320 seconds (cycle time) times DDR (number of patients per day)] divided by 28,800 (available time). Simplified, this is 336,960 (seconds) divided by 28,800 (seconds) = 11.7 FTEs.

HEIJUNKA

Heijunka is another Japanese term that is used to describe the idea of "load-balancing," or an efficient balancing of production over time. Heijunka is a great tool for smoothing out repetitive processes to create a system whereby the amount of time allocated to a resource is commensurate with the amount of time required for the process to be completed in the most efficient way.

Load-balancing issues are most often seen in the medical practice in areas of scheduling, billing, testing, etc. Let's take a quick trip to practice utopia and imagine what a perfectly load-balanced practice would look like:

- All patients would have the same diagnosis.
- All treatments would be exactly the same (and have the same outcome).
- All patients would arrive at the same rate and on time.
- It would take the same amount of time to process each patient visit.
- The bill for all patients would be the same.
- There would only be one payer involved (not an endorsement for a one-payer system!).
- All providers would be equal in their ability to provide quality care.

Unfortunately, this is not ever the case; and, as such, we often see poorly balanced loading within a typical day at the practice. Patients have different chief complaints, and, in fact, some even lie about that. Each encounter is usually approached without prejudice, meaning that treatment options are dependent upon differential diagnoses through evaluation and management efforts. Different types of patients (new, established, visits, procedures, etc.) require different amounts of time, and the actual time it takes for each encounter may vary even more. For the most part, different patients will require the use of different ICD-9 and HCPCS codes, so the bill may be different for each. And with thousand of payers and tens of thousands of insurance products out there, claims will be sent to dozens if not more payers each day. And the beat goes on. Load balancing demands that, for similar processes, a method be established for balancing the process time against the time needed to be efficient. Failing to do this often results in bottlenecks (providers waiting for patients) and backups (patients waiting for providers), reducing efficiency, increasing costs, and negatively effecting patient satisfaction and staff morale.

Using Heijunka in the Practice

As discussed, load-balancing is a necessity for such repetitive processes as scheduling, encounters, billing cycles, procedures and testing, and other such functions. One area that is a common source of pain for many medical practices is phone handling. It is also an area that could use a Heijunka project. So let's take a look at an example that uses Heijunka to solve problems in this area.

Here, we have a practice that is open from 8:00 until 5:00 for patient visits, tests, and procedures. The goal of our study was to take a look at call volume to see what, if any, waste was found and what, if anything, could be done to improve efficiency. To do this, we used a phone system that tracked calls by time and used the results of one month to categorize call volume into hourly compartments. We totaled the number of calls received into the practice per hour and tracked the number of those calls that were actually answered. Those that were not answered went to voice mail and needed to be followed up by a staff member. We then tracked the number of unanswered calls that were successfully returned (meaning that the staff was able to connect with the original caller) on that same day. Answer efficiency was calculated as the calls answered as a percent of all calls, and return efficiency was calculated as the number of calls successfully returned the same day as a percent of all calls. Rework, for our study, was counted as the number of calls in excess of one that had to be made in order to try to connect with the original caller. Figure 27 illustrates a summary of the study results.

In order to get a better (visual) perspective on call volume and patterns, we graphed the data as calls received vs. calls answered (Figure 28). Note the gap in the first hour of the day, lunch time, and the last hour of the day. Remember, the purpose of any study like

Hour	Calls	Answered	Returned	Answer Efficiency	Return Efficiency	Rework
8-9	42	34	3	80.95%	37.50%	11.90%
9-10	36	31	3	86.11%	60.00%	5.56%
10-11	31	28	0	90.32%	0.00%	9.68%
11-12	34	34	0	100.00%	100.00%	0.00%
12-1	51	3	22	5.88%	45.83%	50.98%
1-2	30	26	4	86.67%	100.00%	0.00%
2-3	22	22	0	100.00%	100.00%	0.00%
3-4	26	22	3	84.62%	75.00%	3.85%
4-5	38	21	8	55.26%	47.06%	23.68%

FIGURE 27. Call volume study results.

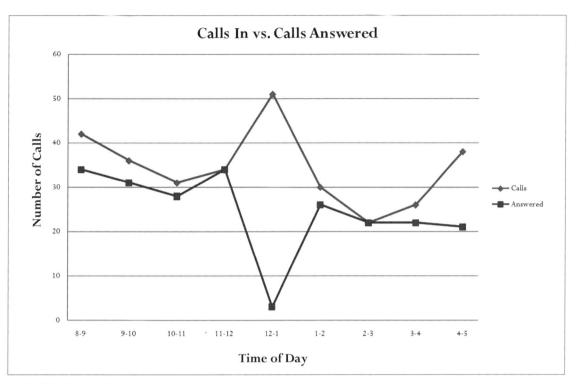

FIGURE 28.   Call volume study graph.

this is to identify variability and to ask why it is happening. In this case, it doesn't require a study: call volume can be associated with patient availability. Early morning is associated with pre-work hours (or drive time), the noon to 1:00 hour is obviously lunch time for many patients (and unfortunately, for all staff members), and the last hour is post-work (or again, drive time).

The goal here is to study (and ultimately improve) the efficiency of the system. Therefore, it's not necessarily the volume of calls per bucket nor even the gap between calls in and calls answered, but rather the amount of rework that is required. And a true Heijunka project is focused on balancing that load such that the amount of rework is minimized by allocating the right resources at the right time. Figure 29 identifies the derivative of the rework effort.

Impact of Load Balancing

Note that approximately 50% of rework effort results from an imbalance in the lunch-time scheduling while over a third occurs during the first and last hour of the day (normally when staff are opening and closing the practice). Objectively, in order to estimate the benefit from any project, it is necessary to create a measurement system that can be tracked

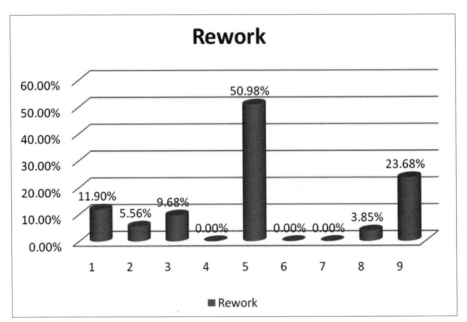

FIGURE 29. **Call volume study rework. The numbers on the horizontal axis represent the hourly intervals for the day (e.g., 1 = 8 to 9 AM, 2 = 9 to 10 AM, etc.).**

and quantified back to the amount resources consumed. In this case, we built a table that measured the impact in those terms (Figure 30).

Notice that we have quantified the amount of time in minutes that result from the lack of balancing staffing requirements for the affected times. Based on this study, waste can be assigned as 7.1 hours per day; and at even a minimum payment of $15 per hour, that translates into $106.50 per day or $27,690 of waste per year. Add to this the effect on patient satisfaction and staff morale, and you have an unnecessary recipe for disaster.

So what do we do? What is the solution? Again, this isn't one of those projects that requires massive brain power, resourcing, or the formation of a formal team or even a charter in order to solve. In fact, using this approach, while the solution may not be easy to implement, it should be pretty clear: reassign staff resources to make sure that calls are handled real-time during the 85% of the rework buckets.

POKA YOKE

Poka Yoke is a Japanese term that means, by practical definition, mistake proofing. In manufacturing, it is a device that prevents incorrect parts from being made or assembled. In service, it is a system that prevents transactional errors, such as not having the same person who deposits the checks also reconcile the checkbook. Poka Yoke, in many cases, goes far-

Calls	Answered	Delta	% of Total	% of Delta	Call-back Volume	Rework Volume	Call Time (minutes)	Rework Time (minutes)
42	34	8	2.58%	8.99%	30	22	54.4	38.1
36	31	5	1.61%	5.62%	19	14	34	23.8
31	28	3	0.97%	3.37%	11	8	20.4	14.3
34	34	0	0.00%	0.00%	-	-	0	-
51	3	48	15.48%	53.93%	182	134	326.4	228.5
30	26	4	1.29%	4.49%	15	11	27.2	19.0
22	22	0	0.00%	0.00%	-	-	0	-
26	22	4	1.29%	4.49%	15	11	27.2	19.0
38	21	17	5.48%	19.10%	65	48	115.6	80.9
310	221	89	28.71%	100.00%	337	248	10.1 hours	7.1 hours

FIGURE 30. Tabular look at rework analysis.

ther than just having a system in place; it also includes some type of audio or visual signal to warn when a mistake is about to occur or has just occurred.

A simple example would be an audible tone that sounds when a caller has been on hold a certain amount of time; say 30 seconds. This prevents the "mistake" of having a patient or other caller sit in the "hold zone" forever, if, for example, the person for whom the call was intended never picked up.

Error-proofing Applications

In the medical practice, there are lots of areas that are candidates for some type of error-proofing since there are lots of opportunities for errors. This is due to the complexity of the business itself. Following are some common areas where Poka Yoke solutions have been applied.

Controlling Patient Flow

In some practices, the physical layout is such that an unescorted patient, after leaving the exam room, can leave the practice building without checking out. This may be due to ingress or egress areas that might be used by staff or emergency exits at locations between treatment or exam rooms and the check-out area. In some cases, doors can be locked, requiring an electronic key, such as a key-card or numerical pad, at the door location. If the doors need to remain unlocked, you can arm them with an alarm system that can be deactivated by staff with a key-code but not by patients. Again, if you can't prevent the event from occurring, you can be notified right away when it occurs.

Numbering Superbill Forms

In order to prevent potential embezzlement and to identify situations when a patient may have slipped out the back, if you do still use a superbill form, these can be sequentially numbered. You can then employ a system such that if a sequenced number is missing, there is a way to investigate real-time.

24-Hour EDI Notification

This actually deals with electronic filing as a solution to A/R problems. If you file claims manually (meaning, you still mail in CMS-1500 forms), it can take several weeks before you find out if there were front-end errors with the claim, such as missing information, incorrect demographics, etc. With the electronic claims process, using an EDI model, the practice is notified either immediately or within 24 hours of these types of errors, giving an almost real-time ability to correct and resubmit these claims.

Patient-in-Room

In busy practices, where there are several providers in several rooms seeing several patients, it is not an uncommon problem to have someone accidentally enter a room while a patient is in a state of undress or actively being examined by a clinician. Some practices have a series of colored plastic flags outside the room with each flag color indicating a state of activity in the room. For example, a red flag indicates the provider is in the room with the patient. A yellow flag would indicate the patient is in the room waiting for the provider. And a green flag might indicate that the room is available. Some practice also use colored lights that are activated from inside the room. The key here is that staff members are trained on and abide by occupation policies. An automatic solution might be to have a motion detector in each room, and when movement is detected, an appropriate warning (such as a colored light) is automatically initiated.

Visit-validation System

While it has been rarely reported, there have been situations where patients have been left in a practice after the office has been closed and everyone has gone home. Sometimes, this has been accidental; and in some cases, it was intentional, and the so-called patient used the opportunity to steal equipment, supplies, and drugs from the practice. One Poka Yoke solution would be to have a system that counts the number of patients in and number of patients out. This is often available through EMR systems and can also be controlled using sequentially numbered superbill forms. While it can be handled manually, through clicker-type counters, the true purpose of Poka Yoke is to have an automated system that has a very high degree of operational confidence.

Controlling Access to Restricted-access Areas

In any medical practice, there are areas that should be off limits to patients and even restricted to certain staff members. This can be controlled through electronic keypads or through the use of key cards. In addition, while some areas may not necessarily be restricted, it is important to know who accessed the area and when it was accessed. Under HIPAA, for example, it is necessary to know who had access to a patient file. This again can be controlled, to physical areas, through the use of keycards that record ID and time to a central computer. For electronic records, this is controlled through password protection schemes that both control and record access. To abide the principles of Poka Yoke, it is important that controls are in place to not only automate this type of error-proofing, but to protect from hacking or bypassing the controls.

5S

Within the TPI toolbox, you can see that some tools are complex, and some are quite simple. Some tools are easy to use, while others are hard. Some tools, on the other hand, are comprised mostly of common sense, and 5S is one of those tools. In fact, if most of us were to function in our business the way our mothers had taught us to function at home, we would all already be experts at 5S. Why? Because 5S is, more than anything else, a means of organizing and picking up after ourselves.

Having said all that, the fact is, 5S is one of the key fundamental tools of process improvement. The reason is simple; the more organized and clean our workspace, the more efficiently we can do our jobs. The simplest example I can think of occurs in most people's showers. The floor area is usually clean and free of debris so we don't trip and fall. The soap, shampoo, conditioner, and other items we commonly use are within easy reach. We normally have a towel hung right outside the shower stall or, in some cases, inside the stall at the back.

Imagine taking a shower and having to leave the shower stall each time you needed a particular item; yet this is how many offices are arranged. The copier is at the opposite end of where the front desk clerk checks in patients, making a copy of everyone's license and insurance card. The printer is in a different room than where the patient records are being prepared for review. Regularly needed items aren't kept in a standard location, and no one knows when they are about to run out.

The point of 5S then, is to work toward a clean, simplified, organized, and standardized workplace that improves the efficiency of the work process. Here are the official 5 Ss along with a (sometimes inadequate) English transliteration; and as you may have guessed by now, the original words are . . . Japanese!

Seiri (Sort)

Separate necessary from unnecessary items, including tools, parts, materials, supplies, and paperwork, and remove the unnecessary items from the work area. I have often seen check-in staff looking for forms that "were just there a minute ago" because the location for those items is not assigned. I have also seen clinicians, in the patient room, wasting time during an exam trying to find a certain diagnostic item or supply, such as an otoscope cover. Once again, this is because there was no assigned location for these items. Seiri is designed to reduce the time wasted looking for necessary items by having a "place for everything and everything in its place" and by removing from the workplace those items that are rarely if ever used.

Seiton (Straighten/Sytematize)

Seiton focuses on arranging the necessary items neatly, providing visual cues to where items should be placed such that accessing everything needed during a normal work process is a no-brainer. The key here is having everything in its right (or logical) place. This might include having the copier right next to the check-in desk so that the check-in clerk needs only to turn to make a copy of intake forms rather than move to the back of the room or even another room. This would also include having the otoscope covers in the same location as the otoscope (hopefully that is also standardized) so that the clinician is not wasting time during the exam. How many times have you checked out of a store with a credit card and there isn't a pen to be found anywhere? In some cases, this may mean putting some items, such as computer work stations, on rolling carts to allow them to be moved from room to room rather than having the provider or nurse go back and forth to a central location to dictate (or scribe) the encounter. Seiton begs that we focus on ergonomics; items that are used most are closest and easiest to reach, and inventoried for replacement when running low.

Seiso (Sweep or Shine)

The basic concept here is to make sure that the work area remains clean. There isn't really much else to say about this as we all know the consequences of clutter: wasted time, effort, and movement. Once you have completed the first two steps, it is normally easier to accomplish this. For example, I make sure that, before I leave my office each day, I have at least sorted through and organized the items I have been working on. I have a set of stackable trays where I prioritize projects or items that I didn't get to today but will have to first thing in the morning. In this way, when I come in the next morning, I don't come into a disorganized mess; my desk is clean and ordered, and I don't spend the first 30 or so minutes trying to figure out what needs to be done first.

Seiketsu (Standardize)

Standardize the first three Ss so that cleanliness, organization, and order are maintained. We will discuss the concept of standardizing processes later (in Chapter 6) but for now, you want to make sure that all of the effort you have put into this tool so far doesn't get lost. And the way that happens is to standardize this around written policies and procedures.

Keeping an area clean, neat, and organized shouldn't be an option; you shouldn't give people a choice on whether they abide by these rules since, by not doing so, it affects the overall efficiency of the entire practice. This requires that every staff member become involved in participating in the process; that each employee has a say in *how* this is to be done rather than *if* it is to be done. This particular S requires discipline and commitment. There are tools and templates that can be developed to assist with auditing the workplace for quality assurance and compliance. One mistake that many practices make is underestimating just how difficult this is to implement and maintain. That is why oversight becomes so important.

Shitsuke (Sustain)

Ensure that the first four Ss continue to be performed on a regular basis. Here, you begin to experience both the benefits, as a result of improved efficiency, and the frustrations, due to the result of human nature. It is pretty common that people not only resist change, but tend to fall back to the traditional ways of doing things even after change has been made and shown to be for the better. The most difficult of the steps is to ensure that this tool remains in place and effective. As I look around my desk right now, as I am writing this chapter, I develop a strong sense of empathy for others involved in trying to maintain this discipline in their workplaces.

Implementing 5S in the Office

If this is going to work, it needs to start at the top. Don't expect employees to take this seriously if, when they walk into the administrator's office, it looks like a train wreck. For me, it's like taking seriously the health advice of a physician who smokes. Contradictions in authority confuse people and make implementation difficult.

You need to also enforce standards. Let the staff who work within the specific environment help to determine how this will work (not whether it will work) so that they are held to their own design. This makes compliance easier than if someone from the outside comes in to tell members of a department how they need to organize their work spaces. When I would complain about how difficult it was to perform a new task, my friend Henry would always respond with, "Practice, practice, practice." And as much as that would really tick me off, it is so true; especially during the initial period when people are the most resistant to change and gravitationally pulled back to their old ways.

One method that I have seen work effectively is to make compliance with 5S standards part of the employee's performance review. In practices that share bonuses with employees, this can be part of the ranking that is used to determine if and how much someone gets. Remember, we are not trying to micromanage anyone's life here, but if one employee's work habits reduce the level of efficiency, then this will eventually create an unnecessary constraint. In too many cases, this introduces a bottleneck, which will ultimately affect the overall profitability of the practice. Ahhh, chaos at its best!

Finally, if you are going to make compliance with 5S part of the performance review, then it is important to also tie some kind of reward (maybe other than part of the bonus calculation) for those employees that both lead out (encouraging others) and do a great job (setting a standard for others).

PRIORITIZATION MATRICES

If you are like me, and like the majority of people out there, you are faced with decisions every day. Some decisions are simple, such as which route to take to work or whether to wear this suit or that one or these shoes or those. Some decisions require more time, like where to go for dinner or what color to choose for a new car or a room in your house. Some decisions take on a more critical tone, such as where to build a new office or whether to invest in large capital projects or whether to even buy a new car at this time. For some decisions, the potential consequences may be minimal; if you paint the wrong color, for a few dollars and a few hours of time, you can just paint another color. For others, the consequences may be more significant, such as the loss of a lot of money if a capital investment doesn't work.

For clinicians, many times the consequences of decisions can mean the difference between life and death or serious long-term debilitation. The point is, nearly every moment of our waking hours is spent in conducting benefit-risk analyses, weighing options, considering the probability of an event (risk), and considering the possible consequences. At times, we do this unconsciously in the blink of an eye; while on the other end of the scale, it is a painstakingly slow and deliberate process that requires pencil and paper, and often a team or committee of people. I have often wondered why, whether unconscious or deliberate, we make bad (or wrong) decisions, and my research points to one key component—emotional involvement. The more we have at risk personally (money, job, family), the more difficult it is to be objective in our decision making.

Have you ever noticed how easy it is for other people to recommend a solution for you when those individuals have little or nothing at stake? Well, many times, their recommendations are the best ones, and the reason is because those making the recommendations *don't* have anything at stake. It's not their risk; it's yours. And that is precisely what a prioritization matrix will do for you—create an objective review of the data to assist with making tough decisions or picking between tough options.

What Is a Priority Matrix?

A priority matrix, sometimes called a decision matrix or Pugh matrix, is a tool that is used to remove anecdotal and subjective components from the decision-making or project-selection process. It helps to translate qualitative information into quantitative data, such as difficulty of implementation; or cost or acceptability; or, in some cases, the political correctness of a decision that results in some action. It is similar to a benefit/risk assessment as, like the Benjamin Franklin-type analysis, it weighs the positive against the negative points.

Unlike the Benjamin Franklin, however, the positive and negative points are weighted to produce numerical values. Priority matrices, in their different forms, are likely the best tools for project selection as well as vetting the sometimes many different good options that come out of a process improvement project team.

Creating the Matrix

In creating the priority matrix, we want to be sure to list all of the criteria necessary to make a decision. For a project, this may include cost, time, doability, resources, risk, regulatory issues, overall effect, etc. For an actionable implementation process, it may include issues around collateral damage, importance of staff buy-in, and the like. The next step is to weigh the importance of each of the criteria using some sort of ranking scale, such as 1 to 10 or 1 to 100. What's critical here is to make sure that the weighting is consistent across the board. Remember, the goal is to build a quantifiable model that makes sense. For example, if cost is the most important factor, it might get a value of 10 (on a 1-to-10 scale with 10 being most important).

Let's say you rate staff buy-in at about a third of the value of the cost of the project. Staff buy-in, would then get a weight of 3 (or 33 on a scale of 1 to 100). Once you have created a weight for each of the criteria, you want to assign a value that represents the benefit/risk factor associated to each criterion. The benefit/risk factors should be rated based on the same scale as the criterion, such as 1 to 10 or 1 to 100. To calculate the overall value of the items within the matrix, the scale value is multiplied by each of the criteria importance values. To determine the winner (or the project or decision that gets the most support), you get the sum of those products, and the highest values should represent the top priority item. For example, while cost has an importance of 10, the benefit/risk relationship might only be a 5 (meaning that the project is associated with an average cost risk). Therefore, the total value associated to this criterion is 50 (importance of 10 times the benefit/risk factor of 5).

Ranking Benefit/Risk Factors

Priority matrices can be quite simple, including only a few basic criteria, or complex, listing and weighing all of the criteria irrespective of the initial perceived importance. In most every matrix, however, we normally see the following three benefit/risk factors associated with the selected criteria: doability, cost, and impact.

Doability (I know that isn't a real word) deals with ease (or difficulty) of implementation. On a scale of 1 to 10, 1 might represent a situation where it would require an organization-wide coordination of effort, such as with a new practice management system or EMR system. If, on the other hand, the team (or individual or small group of individuals) has complete control over implementation, including discretionary ability to make the change and any subsequent adjustment, we might rate doability as a 10 (remember, higher scores mean a higher overall ranking).

Cost deals with the total financial expense (does not include revenue balancing), and in a multi-decisional matrix might relate to each of the potential solutions suggested. Remembering that a higher score usually results in a more favorable view of the criterion, project, or decision point, rating cost is normally accomplished as an inverse relationship to the other benefit/risk components. For example, if it takes an act of Congress to get to the money, you might rate this as a 1, while if it is virtually free or is covered as part of discretionary income, you might rate this as high as a 10.

Benefit/Risk Factors (1 - 10, Agree - Disagree)	Redesign Intake Package	Snail Mail	Internet Access	E-mail as .pdf	Interview on Phone	Weight (1 - 10)
Implemented quickly	8	10	8	9	3	7
Solve the problem completely	8	5	5	5	7	10
Will not negatively impact patient	10	7	10	7	8	6
Will not negatively impact staff	7	10	10	6	3	6
No regulatory risks	8	10	10	10	10	8
Will not compromise quality	10	6	6	8	8	5
Will not cost more than $1,000	10	10	3	7	2	3
Weighted Value	382	362	345	332	283	

FIGURE 31. Complex decision matrix.

The last benefit/risk factor that is commonly seen has to do with impact; what will be the overall impact of this decision/project/change to the organization or department? If the impact is low, for example, or cannot be measured in any meaningful way, it might rate a 1 or a 2. If, on the other hand, it will completely solve the problem or have a huge positive impact on the organization, you might give it a high number such as 9 or 10.

Complex Decision Matrix

As discussed, decision matrices can be simple or complex. Complex matrices might include many different criteria or different levels of criteria, or may even combine both project models as well as decision points. Look at the example in Figure 31, which deals with ways to reduce waiting time between check-in and the exam room.

In this example, we have listed five different solutions to a problem dealing specifically with ways to improve the efficiency of having new patients complete the intake package. These are listed across the top. In the first column, along the left of the table, we have listed the benefit/risk factors and given them a scale rating of 1 to 10, based on level of agreement. For example, for each of the possible solutions, we asked team members to agree or disagree with the statement (albeit truncated) that the potential solutions presents a quick implementation. Notice that snail mail was given a 10 while completing the forms with the patient over the phone was given a 3. If you multiply the benefit/risk factor times the weight, you get the value for that component. In this case, the overall value for snail mail is 70 (10×7) while for interviewing by phone is valued at 21 (3×7). Note that for this practice, cost was defined using a dollar value—will not cost more than $1,000—as opposed to just listing cost as a benefit/risk factor. In this case, it may have been done this way due to a budget limitation that was inflexible and predetermined.

Criteria (1 - 10)	Redesign Intake Package	E-mail as .pdf	Internet Access	Snail Mail	Interview on Phone
Doability (1 = Doable 10 = Not Doable)	8	7	5	9	5
Cost (1 = Very expensive 10 = Cheap)	10	7	4	6	4
Impact (1 = No impact 10 = Solves problem)	5	5	7	7	8
Weighted Value	400	245	140	378	160

FIGURE 32. Simple decision matrix.

Note that, in our example above, after the counts were in and the dust had settled, there emerged two distinct solutions that would be put on the table for further testing: redesigning the intake package and mailing the package out in advance to new patients.

A simple decision matrix, on the other hand, may contain fewer criteria or be more focused on a particular set of solutions. If we were to take the above example and limit it to the three basic benefit/risk factors discussed above, it might look like the example shown in Figure 32.

Note in this table that, rather than having a scale of agreement based on statements, we have scaled the benefit/risk factors on their merit and posed them more as questions than statements. For example, doability is asking the question; how doable is this project considering the overall constraints within the practice? Or with cost, asking the question, "Is this going to cost a lot of money?" In this case, while the overall values are different than above, the results are the same: redesigning the intake package is a no-brainer, while Internet access and phone interviews are beyond consideration at this point.

PARETO

Let's start this discussion by getting the historical issues out of the way. The word *Pareto* is taken from the name of a 19th-century Italian economist by the name of Vilfredo Pareto. Sometime in the late 1800s, he came to the conclusion that 80% of the wealth was controlled by 20% of the population and (voila!) the Pareto effect was born. It was until the 1940s, however, that the idea of using his ideas came to fruition, thanks to a quality engineer by the name of Joseph Juran, who suggested the principle and named it after Pareto.

A Pareto analysis is a statistical technique that is used to identify the limited number of tasks or events that produce the overall effect. It does this by looking at the distribution of data points within a model in order to consider relative control of different factors. A Pareto chart is a graph that illustrates the results of a Pareto analysis. Pareto efficiency, while not necessarily related to our topic here, was developed by the same person and states that in a Pareto-efficient system, certain factors can be changed or manipulated such that the people or components in a system all benefit without any suffering a loss. This is a substitutive model that is used quite often in global economics. As a tool, we are going to discuss the first two components and look at how you can use this tool to assist with problem identification and prioritization of projects and solutions.

The Pareto Rule

In general, the Pareto rule states that 80% of an event can be described by 20% of an action. As Pareto discovered, 80% of the wealth is controlled by 20% of the population. In a medical practice, you might find that approximately 80% of the revenue comes from 20% of your procedure codes or that 20% of your payers control 80% of your payments. From a denial standpoint, you may find that around 80% of the denials are associated with 20% of reason codes. From a project management standpoint, you may find that 80% of the problems can be fixed using only 20% of your resources.

In essence, the Pareto principle, which is also called the vital few principle, tells us that, while not exactly formed in a 80/20 relationship, the vital few factors are normally responsible for 80% of our issues or problems. It is important to note that when we refer to "vital few" or "trivial many," we are referring to a quantitative rather than a qualitative analysis. This means that even those factors that go beyond the 80% rule may still be important (or sometimes critical), they still fall outside of our defined vital few criteria.

Pareto Analysis

A Pareto analysis can be conducted on nearly any set of data that involves two components: factors that create issues and the issues that are the result of those factors. Developing a Pareto analysis means looking at the distribution of these data issue by issue and factor by factor. These are the basic steps involved in conducting the analysis:

1. Collect the data to be reviewed, and organize into either a worksheet or a table.
2. Arrange the rows in descending order based on importance.
3. Calculate, for each row, the percent distribution of the total.
4. Cumulate the percent by adding the prior to the current value.

It is important, however, to differentiate between a frequency distribution table, which can be used for many purposes, and a Pareto analysis, which is used only to associate events to effects.

For example, if you want to analyze the distribution of delay intervals in your waiting room, you would have to define two primary components: what defines a delay (in minutes)

Wait Time (minutes)	Count
1-3	93
4-6	65
7-9	81
10-12	22
13-15	15
16-18	41
19-21	26
22-24	34
25-27	31
28-30	21
31+	17

FIGURE 33. Base table for wait-time calculations.

Wait Time (minutes)	Count	Percent
1-3	93	20.85%
4-6	65	14.57%
7-9	81	18.16%
10-12	22	4.93%
13-15	15	3.36%
16-18	41	9.19%
19-21	26	5.83%
22-24	34	7.62%
25-27	31	6.95%
28-30	21	4.71%
31+	17	3.81%

FIGURE 34. Frequency distribution table for wait time analysis.

and the intervals that you want to measure. Let's say you define an acceptable wait time as up to 30 minutes. Therefore, anything beyond this is considered excessive. You could use a distribution table to identify the percent of events that occurs during each interval period of minutes after the initial 30 minutes of wait time. First, you could record the total number of minutes and create a set of buckets for excessive wait time, such as 1 to 3 minutes, 4 to 6 minutes, 7 to 10 minutes, 11 to 14 minutes, 15 to 18 minutes, etc. You would then create a table that showed how many times each of those buckets was recorded, as shown in Figure 33.

The next step is to assign a percent to each. This is done by dividing the individual count by the total count for the event; in this case, 446 (Figure 34).

In a Pareto analysis, you would now add a column that cumulates the percent to identify at which point you reach the 80% mark, as shown in Figure 35.

Note that while the cumulate percent gives you interesting data, it doesn't have any particular value with respect to cause and effect. In this table, we can see that around 80% of excessive wait time falls somewhere between 19 and 24 minutes. But what about wait time above 24 minutes? That may be even more important with regards to patient satisfaction, which, if you associated to this, could make this a viable candidate for a Pareto analysis. In fact, you don't, and therefore this is simply a frequency table. And while the information is important, it does not follow the Pareto principle in that it does not identify the potential for cause and effect.

Wait Time (minutes)	Count	Percent	Cumulative Percent
1-3	93	20.85%	20.85%
4-6	65	14.57%	35.43%
7-9	81	18.16%	53.59%
10-12	22	4.93%	58.52%
13-15	15	3.36%	61.88%
16-18	41	9.19%	71.08%
19-21	26	5.83%	76.91%
22-24	34	7.62%	84.53%
25-27	31	6.95%	91.48%
28-30	21	4.71%	96.19%
31+	17	3.81%	100.00%

FIGURE 35. Wait time analysis table showing cumulative frequency distribution.

Reason	Count	Percent	Cumulative Percent
Intake forms	122	42.36%	42.36%
Physician late	44	15.28%	57.64%
Overbooked	38	13.19%	70.83%
Walk-in	27	9.38%	80.21%
Patient late	23	7.99%	88.19%
Parking	17	5.90%	94.10%
Emergency	11	3.82%	97.92%
Weather	6	2.08%	100.00%

FIGURE 36. Frequency distribution table for reasons patients give for being late.

Let's take the example and move it into Pareto territory. Let's say that instead of defining time blocks, you want to know the factors (or reasons) behind excessive wait time. During your brainstorming session, you came up with eight primary factors that the team believed were behind excessive waiting time and then selected a random population of patients that exceeded the 30-minute criterion to determine which factor could be attributed to that wait event. Figure 36 displays those results.

Note that the data have been sorted in descending order. Here we can see that intake forms, physicians being late, overbooking patients, and attending to walk-in patients are

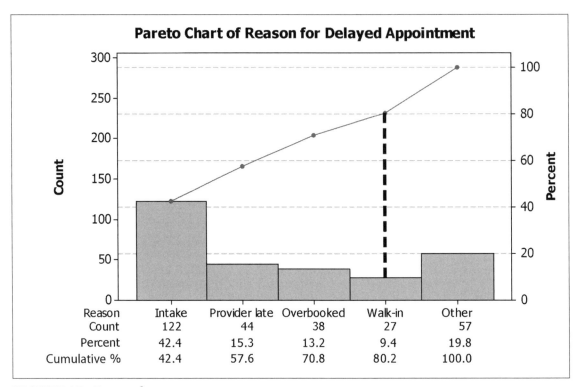

FIGURE 37. Pareto chart.

the most common factors (the vital few) affecting excessive wait time. While the others do have an impact and are in fact important, from a standpoint of prioritizing solutions and resources, you focus on the top 80%, which in this case, consists of the four factors mentioned above.

Pareto Charts

One of the most powerful aspects of a Pareto analysis is the Pareto chart. A Pareto chart is a graph that is designed to assist with visualizing the data by comparing two data simultaneously: the percent contribution of each individual factor and the cumulative impact of all of the factors. This is done in three steps
1. Plot a bar graph that shows the percent contribution of each of the factors in the table.
2. Plot a line graph, on the same chart, that shows the cumulative effect for each factor in successive order.
3. Mark the 80% point on the x-axis.

When complete, a Pareto chart can take a table like the one above and visualize the results as shown in Figure 37.

Zip Code	Count	Percent	Cumulative
33430	6228	15.63%	15.63%
33424	6058	15.20%	30.83%
33212	6009	15.08%	45.91%
33409	4912	12.32%	58.23%
33429	4288	10.76%	68.99%
33417	4061	10.19%	79.18%
33405	2944	7.39%	86.57%
33431	742	1.86%	88.43%
33436	673	1.69%	90.12%
33727	407	1.02%	91.14%
32614	322	0.81%	91.95%
33804	165	0.41%	92.36%
33882	151	0.38%	92.74%
99999	2894	7.26%	100.00%

FIGURE 38. **Patient origin by zip code.**

The beauty of this is that it communicates the purpose of the analysis to everyone involved in a project without the clutter of a frequency table or the need to explain the calculations. We can see very clearly here that the intake forms have the greatest overall effect on wait time, and this moves the process forward into a cause-and-effect session that can be used for rapid and effective improvement.

One salient point to note is the importance of orders of magnitude regarding the Pareto analysis. A rule of thumb says that, within the group of 80%, the most important factors diminish when the subsequent is less than 50% of the prior.

Let's look at another example of a Pareto analysis that is common in many medical practices, that of patient origin by zip code. The reason practices conduct this kind of study is to get an idea of market area, particularly as it pertains to market share for existing and new services. The reason that it is considered a good candidate for a Pareto analysis is because the density of patient origin can be used to determine the effect on such things as marketing dollars and effort, feasibility of new services or expanding existing services, market penetration in developing communities, etc.

Figure 38 is the table that was compiled from a two-year study of patient origin by zip code.

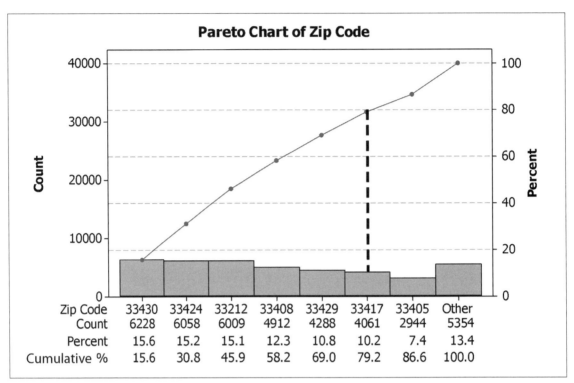

FIGURE 39. Pareto chart of patient origin by zip code.

While there were many more zip codes involved in the study, for the purpose of brevity, I compiled the remaining 50 or so into a category labeled as 99999. Here, we can see that the 80% mark falls right after zip code 33417 and our Pareto chart (Figure 39) illustrates this.

Here we can see that the most influential factors (zip codes) for our practice that affect revenue (or volume or charges, etc.) come from approximately six zip codes. If we were looking to establish some type of linear relationship between marketing effort and origin, we would look at directing 80% of our marketing efforts (or dollars) to those six locations.

One salient point to note about Pareto charts is that they help to identify a rule of thumb that is used to increase the granularity of factoring, even within the 80%. This rule says that when the order of magnitude of a factor drops by more than 50% of the prior factor, you have found the more important contributors to the problem or issue. Take a look at the following Pareto chart (Figure 40) that shows the reason codes reported during a six-month period for a medical practice.

Note that even though there are five reason codes that make up the top 80% reported, reason code 27 dominates by several orders of magnitude over the next reason code (96) listed. In fact, reason code 96 is only about half as contributory as code 27, and therefore,

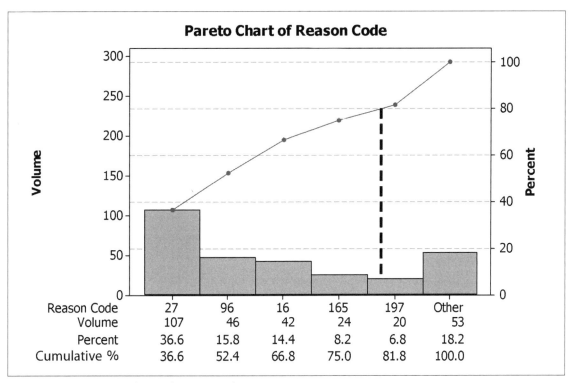

Pareto Chart of Reason Code

Reason Code	27	96	16	165	197	Other
Volume	107	46	42	24	20	53
Percent	36.6	15.8	14.4	8.2	6.8	18.2
Cumulative %	36.6	52.4	66.8	75.0	81.8	100.0

FIGURE 40. **Pareto chart of reason codes.**

if resources are at a premium, the practice would concentrate its efforts first and foremost on resolving the issues that created a denial due to reason code 27.

MSA DRILLDOWN

MSA stands for Measurement System Analysis. It may seem a bit convoluted that we have to measure the systems that we use to measure the systems, but think about the importance of accurate data. If the data you are collecting are not accurate, then the results you arrive at will also be inaccurate. And bad data almost always ends up as bad business decisions, something none of us can afford to make.

An MSA drilldown, as a tool, is a structured approach to checking the quality of data. It is based on the principle that you should not be using data if: 1) you don't know where it came from; and 2) you can't validate its accuracy. In this sense, the MSA drilldown helps to challenge the "pedigree" of the data.

As an example, some practice management and/or EMR systems measure the amount of time it takes a patient to go through the visit cycle each step at a time. As a result, you may decide to use that data to analyze the visit cycle in increments, such as check-in to exam room, time with the provider, etc. Before you undertake this project, however, it would be prudent to assess the accuracy of the measurements being recorded by your system. How would you do this? You would start by randomly selecting some patient visits and following the patient around with a stopwatch. Then compare the time you record with the time reported by the system. If it is on the mark, you can conduct your study with confidence in the data. If it is not, then you will need to make the appropriate adjustments, if possible. If you can't change the measurement system for your PMS or EMR system, then you would need to conduct the study more manually or by using a different automated method.

There are other issues that the MSA drilldown can address, such as how we define measurement points. For example, if we want to measure average waiting room time, we would want to record, for a random set of patients, the amount of time they waited in the waiting room; seems simple enough. But we have some issues to define first, like what constitutes the start of the wait time? Is it when they actually enter the office, or does the time start after they check in? I have seen, in some busy practices, patients wait several minutes before the check-in process is complete. In some cases, patients indicate their arrival on a sign-in sheet and then sit in the waiting room until called to the check-in station to be processed. Do we start the clock upon arrival, sign-in, or check-in? And we may even want to define further what constitutes check-in: is it when the process starts or when it is finished? We should consider how this affects the patients (our customer). While we may not consider wait time to start until after check-in, the patient may be mentally recording the time from the moment he or she walks in the door.

Figure 41 shows one method to map the data measurement process. As with other graphs, charts, and diagrams, visualizing the process steps always makes the job easier.

Notice here that we look at the definitions for both start and stop time, considering the different issues that affect our definition of how the data will be measured. It may seem a bit trivial at first but consider that there may be different people taking measurements at different times. While there may or may not be a "correct" method, it is critically important that it is consistently applied across the board and that it can be defended as accurate and appropriate.

BRAINSTORMING

Brainstorming is one of the key tools behind root cause analysis. As mentioned, many practices get to the correlation phase of process improvement; they know something is wrong and may even know what it is, but they never get to the root cause of the problem. If you don't know that "why" of a problem, it is highly unlikely that you will ever be able to fix it.

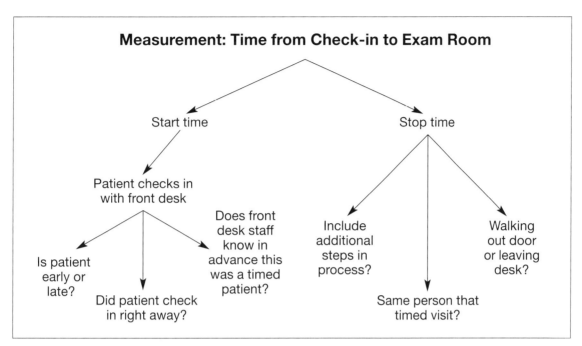

FIGURE 41. **Data measurement process.**

Using brainstorming techniques, you can get to the root cause of a problem; and in many cases, you are surprised by just how many possible causes there can be.

In order for a brainstorming session to be successful, there are some steps that are important for structuring the session. For one, the problem must be both well defined and familiar; well defined in order to be ballistic in our thought process. Broad issues like, "Our A/R is too high" results in broad responses, like, "It takes too long to get paid," which are of little or no value in getting to the root of the issue. Being more specific, such as, "Collections from patients for their responsibility has decreased over the past year," can stimulate more specific ideas, such as, "We don't have a collection script common to all employees." Considering this, it is important that the problem is not too complex or multifaceted. Keeping is simple—not in respect to the nature of the issue but rather the focus of the problem—becomes an important factor, and, as such, time should be taken to ensure that the problem statement is appropriate for a brainstorming session.

In more complex issues, it is often effective to break the problem down into smaller sub-groups. Size of the group is important; too many people, and you will never get through this. Too few, and the ideas and possible causes to a problem may be limited with real causes not being discovered. My experience is that there should be fewer than 3 or more than 10 people within the group. Makeup of the group is also important. Be sure to have process owners and experts available, as in many cases, the folks who are in decision-making positions actually don't have a clue as to what happens on the floor of the practice. For financial issues, have the financial people available. If it deals with patient flow, have the check-in and subclinical staff available. For issues that deal with billing and collection, have your coding and billing staff present. In some cases, such as a solo or small practice, everyone may be involved, and that's OK as long as someone is in control.

Which brings me to my next point: have a facilitator. While brainstorming sessions may sometimes feel like a free-for-all, without facilitation and control, many relevant ideas may be missed, passed over, or never even expressed. Remember, efficiency is what we are all about, and having an efficient process to create an efficient process is, well, very efficient. Finally, because it is often difficult to get things started, someone should have a set of lead questions ready. For example, if A/R is on the table, maybe start with a question like, "How well are we doing with regards to collecting patient co-pay at check-in?," or if it has to do with patient cycle time, you might start with something like, "Do we know whether new patients complain about waiting time more than existing patients do?" The idea is to kick-start the process but not to control it or steer it in any direction.

Rules for Brainstorming

In addition to structuring the steps, there are some basic rules that should be considered in order to maximize both the efficiency and results of the session. To begin, the problem statement should be in the form of a question. For example, if the problem is returning patient phone calls in a timely manner, instead of saying, "It takes too long to return patient phone calls," we might instead ask, "Why does it take so long to return patient phone calls?" Remember, the goal is to come up with possible reasons as to "why" something is happening (or not happening, for that matter).

When responding, make sure that only one person responds at a time. Have you ever been in one of those meetings (or a family dinner), where every time you open your mouth to say something, someone else blurts something ahead of you? Well, that is very frustrating and results in either negativity or a slump in participation. I like to put, in large letters on the white board, OPAT, which stands for "One Person At a Time." One effective way to accomplish this is to start at one point and go around in some orderly fashion, like around the table or up and down rows. For this to be most effective, everyone must participate verbally, even if all they say is "Pass." Keep going in this order until everyone has passed, and hopefully you will have exhausted all possible ideas. You always want to have a recorder, either a person or equipment, that records every idea, suggestion, cause . . . whatever. Not recording someone's response can create disappointment or embarrassment and, ultimately, resignation from the process. If there are lots of people or ideas are coming quickly, you may want to have more than one person recording those responses. They can be written on sticky notes and stuck to a wall, or written down on an easel (flip chart) or white board. My preference is the easel pad because the responses can be seen clearly by everyone, and the pages can be retained for future reference. If you use a white board, be sure to take a picture of the contents before erasing it and moving on. In this phase of the process improvement cycle, we are after quantity, not quality. While there is always levity regarding some responses, it is important there be absolutely no criticism or mocking of any response.

During the brainstorming session, the purpose is not to judge the quality of the response—that comes later—but rather to get as many ideas as possible. When using brainstorming for initial phases, such as project selection, or for later phases, such as prioritization of improvements, you will often be surprised at how what initially appears as a "silly" idea turns out to be the best. Having said this, it doesn't mean that there can't be any discussion. For example, questions to clarify a concept, topic, or idea are perfectly acceptable and will often result in generation of additional ideas. It also results in piggybacking—building on other's ideas.

Negative Brainstorming

Sometimes, brainstorming doesn't produce the results you would like, which is a high quantity of results. When this happens, you can try what is called negative brainstorming. It is pretty much what the name says: brainstorming the negatives, or opposites, of the issue in question. For example, you may have hit a wall regarding the question of how to improve the visit cycle. A negative brainstorming question might be something like, "What could be done to really mess up our visit cycle process?" Responses might be to overbook all slots, not allow enough time for each visit, or not have any way to know if a patient has entered the office. For a question such as how to improve the billing cycle, negative brainstorming might elicit ideas like, "Don't update our coding books," or "Don't bother to verify insurance," or "Let the billing people determine what code should be applied to the visit." For A/R issues, someone might respond, "Never write off outstanding balances." The idea is to look at the issue from the back side and then just reverse the logic.

Some Keys to Success

For a brainstorming session to be successful, whether for root cause, project selection, building priority matrices, or just creating a process improvement idea, don't limit thinking or imagination. So often, I have seen what should have been a very successful process spiral into the dirt because someone in the room was a dream-squasher. Try this: if you don't have something encouraging or constructive to say, then say nothing (or, of course, "Pass," if it's your turn). Wait until all ideas have been presented—until everyone has passed—to begin combining, reviewing, and eliminating ideas for feasibility and impact. You may even want to wait to do this at a subsequent meeting. Use affinity diagramming for large lists—a tool that is used to group ideas into major buckets, or categories, based on criteria established by the group. Sometimes, multi-voting or prioritization matrices can be created to further define categories of ideas based on different criteria, such as cost, doability, and potential for creating viable solutions. This is necessary when the purpose of the session is to find ideas for immediate implementation. Finally, the facilitator should build a consensus on choices. There are three levels to consensus building. First, no one opposes the idea or solution outright. Second, all team members can support the idea even though it may not be popular or a first choice. And third, no solution is defined as undoable, even when not everyone likes it.

MULTI-VOTING

Irrespective of the specific technique, there are some basic rules and steps that should be considered. The first and most obvious is to come up with a list of ideas, solutions, issues, etc. The next is to categorize, organize, or otherwise structure the list of items in some logical fashion. When a final list has been tallied, the team begins to vote on each item. In a single-round procedure, the initial votes are often cast "in the blind," or by secret ballot. Each member can vote one time for as many different items such that a member may vote for all items or no items based on his or her own discretion. Once the voting is complete, a tally is conducted, and the results are visually posted. One common method is to place a dot or hash mark next to each item as it receives a vote so everyone can see the progress. Once the initial vote is in, depending on the number of items, you may want to make a "short list" and vote again; this constitutes multi-round voting.

A good method to determine if this will be necessary is to decide ahead of time how many ideas can be reasonably considered. Let's say you have 10 ideas on the board and you want to eliminate half; in essence, set a limit of five ideas that you believe can be managed by your team. Once the votes are in, you simply take the top five. If there is a tie, you have a vote-off between those tied items. With larger lists, say as many as 100 ideas, you may want to set up an initial filtering process that would require each item to get a certain number of votes. One way to do this is to take the number of voters (team members) and divide by three; that would be the minimum number of votes required to keep an item on the board. In there are 10 team members, then an item needs at least three votes to remain in consideration. Using our list of 100 as an example, let's say you have set a limit of 10 ideas. The initial vote brings you to 30. You would then have a second vote (and if necessary, a third or more) to further cull the list. Again, in this case, the top 10 would remain with vote-offs occurring for tied items.

It may sound a bit confusing, but in reality, it is a logical method that is designed to narrow the options to a manageable size, and multi-voting is a very effective method to accomplish this goal.

General Rules for Multi-Voting

As a practical matter, you can't work on everything at once or use every suggestion, hence the purpose of multi-voting in the first place. With larger teams, you may want to limit the number of votes for team members. For example, for a list of 10 things, you assign three votes per member. For a list of 20 things, you would assign five votes per member. For a list of 30 items, you would assign eight votes per member. For larger lists, you could use an affinity diagram strategy to isolate ideas into buckets and then multi-vote a few from each bucket.

Other alternatives include burning votes; this is where you allow each person to use multiple votes for ideas they particularly like. You can also weight the votes. Using sticky dots or small sticky notes, assign descending values to ideas based on priority, and then add the values on the votes that are posted to the chart.

As discussed, multiple rounds of voting are also quite successful. For example, in round 1, everyone votes for their top five ideas. In round two, everyone gets just three votes to pick from the top five vote-getters in round 1. Remember, there aren't any hard-and-fast rules except to be flexible enough to get to your goal without sacrificing the quality of the project or the solution.

ASSUMPTION BUSTING

Assumption busting is a great tool when people are having a hard time coming up with solutions. It encourages thinking outside the box by opening our minds to ideas outside of our normal comfort zone. Sounds pretty eclectic, but it's actually quite basic and can even be fun.

For example, if we are looking at improving the visit cycle, we would start with assumptions, expressed through the ideas of our patients, such as the patients don't care how long they wait; or patients are happy as long as they are sitting in the exam room (the second waiting room!); or we assume that new patient paperwork can be completed in 10 minutes irrespective of the literacy or linguistics of the patient. If we are looking at the billing cycle, assumptions might be that front-end scrubbers are useless or, on the contrary, they are perfect; both of which are poor assumptions. In selecting an EMR system, we might make the assumption that EMR systems always select the right code or that modifiers are always options. Regarding A/R, we might make the usually false assumption that appeals always cost more than they return.

The key is to test each assumption against a number of standards, the least of which is reality.

HYPOTHESIS TESTING

Hypothesis testing is, for the most part, a statistical process that is used to determine the significance and/or validity of our data. It refers to the process of using statistical analysis to determine if the observed differences between two or more samples are due to random chance (as stated in the null hypothesis) or to true differences in the samples (as stated in the alternate hypothesis). A null hypothesis is a stated assumption that there is no difference in parameters (mean, median, variance, etc.) for two or more populations or, in some cases, two samples. The alternate hypothesis is a statement that the observed difference or relationship between two populations is real and not the result of chance or an error in sampling.

In hypothesis testing, we use a variety of statistical tools to analyze the data and, ultimately, to fail to reject the null hypothesis. From a practical point of view, finding statistical evidence that the null hypothesis is false allows you to reject the null hypothesis and accept the alternate.

For example, suppose we are looking at collection percentages for a particular doctor and we want to know whether the collection percent for that doctor (i.e., 45%) is different from that of his peer group. The null hypothesis [H(o)] would be that there is no difference and would be stated as H(o) = .45. The alternative hypothesis [H(a)] has two options: the collection percent is less than the peer group or it is more than the peer group. If we are interested in only one of these directions, this would be referred to as a one-tail test since we are looking to see the probability of the data falling within either the left or right tail of the distribution. In this case, the scenarios would be either H(a) > .45 or H(a) < .45. If we didn't care whether the value was more or less (we only care if it is different), we would refer to this as a two-tail test since we are looking at the probability that the value being tested would appear in either the left or the right tail.

What sort of data would we need to reject H(o)? Well, the value of .45 would have to be significantly different than that of the comparison group, and again significance is measured the probability of occurrence within the tail or tails of the distribution. Significance is defined by the probability of chance that we are willing to accept. For example, if the collection rate of .45 occurred in less than 5% of all of the other doctors sampled, and we set the critical value at 5%, then we would say that this doctor's collection amount is significantly different; or in the process of hypothesis testing, we would reject the null hypothesis that his collection percent was the same as the peer group. We could, for example, have a higher level of critical test value, such as falling below 1%. In this case, then, we would have accepted the null hypothesis that the collection percent was statistically the same as the peer group.

Within every test, there is a chance of making a mistake regarding our prediction and the lower the p-value (and consequently the larger the confidence interval), the lower the risk of an error. In hypothesis testing, there are two types of errors: type I errors and type II errors. In a type I error, we run the risk of rejecting the null hypothesis when it is, in fact, true, such as declaring that 45% is not the same as the peer group when it actually is the same. In a type II error, we run the risk of accepting the null when it isn't true, such as declaring that the 45% is the same as the peer group average when in fact it is not. Again, in both cases, risk can be controlled based on certain parameters.

Let's look at an example of a real application of a hypothesis test in the form of a legal case involving elections. Nicolas Caputo, a democrat and the Elections Commissioner for Essex County, New Jersey, sets the ballot order (who comes first and so on on a given ballot) based on a coin toss. Landing on heads gives that party top billing on the ballot. After 41 elections, democrats were at the top (won the toss) 41 times. The republicans were pretty upset and claimed that the toss was rigged and based their claim on statistics—a hypothesis test. The null hypothesis was that, with a fair coin, it would land on heads 50% of the time. Therefore, H(o) = .5. The alternate hypothesis is that the coin would land on heads more or less than 50% of the time, making H(a) ≠ .5. An initial test is done to determine the 95% confidence interval for this proportion based on 40 tosses of a coin. What we want to know is this: assuming that the probability is 50%, for what range would we expect to see a heads appear 95% of the time? The answer is 33.8% to 66.2%. This means that if, in 100 different attempts, we flipped a fair coin 40 times, we would expect that in at least 95 of those attempts, the heads would appear somewhere between 33.8% and 66.2% of the time. Another way to look at it is this: if heads showed up fewer than 14 times or more than 22 times in 40 tosses, I would suspect that this was not a fair coin as these values would fall within the area of the tail that indicated that the probability this would happen is less than 5%. We have set our critical value at 5% here, meaning that if the probability of the result is below 5% (the p-value), we reject the null hypothesis that this is a fair coin.

So if he really did toss a fair coin, what is the probability that, out of 41 tosses, it would land on heads 40 times? It is approximately 0.0000000018%, well below our critical p-value of 5%. In this case, we reject the null hypothesis and accept that this is not a fair coin. By the way, the New Jersey Supreme Court agreed that this was "beyond a reasonable doubt."

Since hypothesis testing is steeped in statistical analyses and testing and that is not the purpose of this chapter, I am going to avoid the technical mathematics and focus on applications to the medical practice. But first, let's examine, perhaps, the most common example of hypothesis testing available to us: our system of justice. In the United States, the law states that a person is innocent until proven guilty. And in a situation in which a person is accused of a crime, it is the burden of the accuser to provide enough evidence to prove his or her case beyond "a shadow of a doubt." In statistical terms, "shadow of a doubt" would be represented by the probability that the person committed a crime is between the tails of the distribution, discussed above, or greater than the critical probability that the event didn't occur.

In our hypothetical criminal case, a person is accused of a crime and the "innocent until proven guilty" is equivalent to the null hypothesis; we assume innocence unless there is compelling evidence to cause us to disagree with that assumption. Therefore, H(o) = innocent. The alternate hypothesis is that the person is guilty (or better stated as "not innocent"), and while we may never know with 100% certainty whether a person is really innocent or guilty, our system is based on the process of rejecting the null (innocent), which results in a guilty verdict. So, the jury hears the testimony of the two sides and retires to deliberate with the goal of either accepting the null hypothesis, which would result in a verdict of innocent, or rejecting the null hypothesis (which would involve accepting the alternate hypothesis), which would result in a verdict of guilty. Both conditions cannot be met (both innocent and not innocent cannot occur simultaneously).

As stated above, there is always the chance of making a mistake. Rejecting the null (finding the defendant guilty) when he or she is actually innocent is a type I error. Accepting the null (finding the defendant not guilty) when he or she is actually guilty is a type II error. This is often represented in a table like the one shown in Figure 42.

Hypothesis testing boils down to two things: what is the probability that something happened purely by chance, and what probability are you willing to accept before you declare that event as significant. There are dozens of different hypothesis tests that can be

The Truth	The Verdict	
	Defendant <u>is not</u> guilty: H_0 accepted	Defendant <u>is</u> guilty: H_0 rejected
Defendant <u>is</u> <u>not</u> guilty: H_0 true	Justice is served	(I) An innocent man is convicted Type I Error
Defendant <u>is</u> guilty: H_0 false	(II) A guilty man is set free Type II Error	Justice is served

FIGURE 42. **Example of type I and type II errors.**

applied depending on a myriad of parameters, such as the distribution of the data, how many different items are being compared, the size of the sample, whether it is a proportion being tested, or the difference between two means. What is important here is to know that we can't always determine the significance of a value, the difference between two values, or the relative truth of a statement without the tool of hypothesis testing.

References

1. King MS, Lipsky MS, Sharp L. Expert agreement in current procedural terminology evaluation and management coding. *Arch Intern Med*. 2002;162:316-320.
2. Gruber J, Rodriguez D. How much uncompensated care do doctors provide? *Journal of Health Economics*. 2007;26:1151–1169.
3. Temkin BD. Customers will get more attention in 2005: survey of NA firms identifies customer experience priorities. Forrester Research White Paper, March 15, 2005.
4. Kano N, Seraku N, Takahashi F, Tsuji S. Attractive quality and must-be quality [in Japanese]. *Journal of the Japanese Society for Quality Control*. 1984;14(2):39-48.

SIX

Deployment Platforms

You never change something by fighting the existing reality.
To change something, build a new model that makes
the existing model obsolete.

— R. BUCKMINSTER FULLER

S O MANY TIMES I HAVE COME ACROSS tools that were unrecognizable. When I had my air conditioner replaced, the repair technician had a set of tools that, frankly, were as foreign to me as a box stretcher (that's a joke, actually). In order to effectively use the tools discussed in the prior chapter, we need to be able to learn how to deploy them and to do so in a way that optimizes their use. I hear practices discuss new technology, and they may mention that they are going to be "deploying" a new electronic medical record (EMR) system, or they speak of "deployment" as it refers to a new clinical procedure or capital improvement project. In this sense, the word "deployment" means the process of putting something (a project, program, clinical procedure, etc.) into use systematically or logically. A platform refers to a model, of sorts, that is used as a means of managing the tools used to deploy the above-mentioned project, program, or procedure. So, for our purposes here, then, a deployment platform is a means of putting the tools for Total Practice Improvement (TPI) into use systematically and/or logically.

There are many deployment platforms that are in use for Lean, Six Sigma, and Lean Six Sigma projects. And, I suspect, more are on the way. Since there seems to be a bit of homogeneity with regards to purpose and plan, it behooves us to limit our discussion to those that seem to have gained the greatest popularity while, at the same time, allow for the greatest stratification across project paradigms. In this chapter, we are going to discuss the following platforms:

- DMAIC
- PDSA/PDCA
- IDEA

- FOCUS
- A3
- Kaizen

While each of these will contain redundancies when compared with the others, each has its own pros and cons when it comes to the deployment decision. For example, PDCA is a basic model that is quite effective in smaller organizations or for smaller projects. A3 is more focused on problem solving rather than formal process improvement. DMAIC is likely the most formal and resource-intensive of the platforms.

After investigation, you will find that all of these platforms (plus the majority of other platforms) have several features in common. First, they require that the issue or the problem be logically defined. Remember, project selection is based on need, doability, affordability, and correctability. Sometimes, defining the issue is simple; it's in your face, or in some cases, it is mandated by the higher-ups. Often times, it requires brainstorming and/or development of priority matrices to pick the "best of the bunch" when multiple projects are being considered. The second step is to quantify the issue and create the benchmarks. This can be accounts receivable (A/R) days, average provider compensation, utilization of certain procedure codes or modifiers, fee schedules, and a host of other measurements surrounding the specific issue or project. An analysis and understanding of the data are critical components and are either incorporated into this step, or, as in the case of DMAIC, reduced to two individual steps. Root cause analysis is not only common to each platform but perhaps the most important tool of all; without it, we always end up just short of the information we need in order to find a workable solution.

So many practices that I have spoken to or worked with get through the project selection and measurement phases, and then the project dies because they never get to this step. It should go without saying that if we knew the "why" that something was happening, we wouldn't be too far from the "how" to fix it. Yet the overwhelming majority of practices, after identifying and quantifying the problem, simply don't work through this important step in any deployment model. Once the "why" and "how" have been thoroughly delineated, it is time to begin to develop solutions. This is always best handled as a brainstorming session (or series of brainstorming sessions).

Process owners, administration, stakeholders, and often patients will make up the team that begins to identify possible solutions to the problem. As part of this phase, developing ways to test and implement the solutions should be planned in advance and given the resources necessary to be effective. The final phase in most deployment platforms is that of validation and follow-up. For many, after having committed time, money, personnel, and other resources, knowing whether or not the "fix" works should be of paramount importance. If it doesn't, then rethink and rework the model. If it does, then plan for a way to continue to measure the effects of your changes, and make the new, improved process a part of the standard operating procedure of the practice.

DMAIC: THE KING OF PROCESS IMPROVEMENT

> *Don't fear failure so much that you refuse to try new things. The saddest summary of life contains three descriptions: would have, should have, could have.*
>
> —LOUIS BOONE

Whole books have been written just on DMAIC, as well they should. DMAIC is truly the king of process improvement and the major driver in Six Sigma projects. As stated above, however, Six Sigma is not a very good model for medical practices, and therefore, many assume that neither is DMAIC. Nothing could be further from the truth! DMAIC, from an exhaustive review, is, in its entirety, a beast. It is big, bulky, time consuming, and, at times, irreverent. DMAIC can open a Pandora's box of overwhelming forks in the road and options to pursue that, once released, can quickly consume a project with tangential lines of other potential projects until it chokes the life out of the team. Whew! That's a lot! But wait, there's more . . . DMAIC is also one of the most versatile and polymorphic platforms we have. Because it encompasses virtually every phase and step of every other platform (i.e., A3, PDSA, FOCUS, IDEA, etc.), it holds endless possibilities irrespective of the iterative processes we encounter.

To be more specific, no one project encompasses all of the components in DMAIC; some projects make use of many of the components, and most others will depend upon some of the components. Therefore, DMAIC is polymorphic; it can be applied to pretty much any process improvement or problem-solving situation. In conclusion, Six Sigma is nothing without DMAIC but DMAIC can function quite well outside of Six Sigma. If you will take the time to become an expert in the DMAIC platform, you will be able to address every problem at nearly every level imaginable.

What Is DMAIC?

As stated above, DMAIC is a polymorphic, conclusive, and transparent process improvement platform. It consists of five phases, as follows:

- Define
- Measure

- Analyze
- Improve
- Control

Following, we will examine, in a good deal of detail, each of these phases, including for each the goals and objective and the steps and tools required to make it work. Just remember, not everything discussed here will apply to all (or even any) of your projects, so as you go through this section, take notes regarding which tools, steps, and components are most applicable to the size of and resources available to your organization.

Define

This is the "contract" phase of the project. We are determining exactly what we intend to work on and estimating the impact to the business. In the Define phase, we want to:

- Define the business case;
- Understand the customer;
- Define the process;
- Manage the project; and
- Gain project approval.

The Define toolbox consists of the following tools:

- Project Charter
- Stakeholder Analysis
- SIPOC (suppliers, inputs, process, output, and customers)
- As-is Process Map
- Voice of the Customer (VOC)
- Kano Model
- Critical-to-Quality (CTQ) Tree

Each of these has already been discussed in some detail in Chapter 5, The TPI Toolbox.

The Project Charter

The project charter is a formalized way to set the stage for beginning a DMAIC project. It helps to bring order and perspective to the project and is used to determine the direction the project will take. The key components of the project charter are:

- Business case
- Problem statement
- Scope of the project

- Goals and objectives of the project
- Realistic and achievable milestones
- Clearly defined roles and responsibilities

Using these tools, you will find that maintaining focus on the project at hand will be easier, and it will help to keep people motivated in the right areas.

Business Case. The business case is a high-level articulation of the area of concern. It answers two primary questions:

- What is the business motivation for considering the project?
- What is the general area of focus for the improvement effort?

A successful business case is achieved through good interviewing techniques; after all, understanding the nature of the issue and how it relates to the company is critical. It is not uncommon, when people are new at this, to become verbose when brevity and clarity are the order of the day. A good rule is to use as few words as possible to effectively communicate your point but not so few words that the issue is not clearly articulated. Be careful not to use a lot of technical jargon as the business case will likely be read by people not directly involved in the project.

Here are a few business case examples:

- An internal medicine practice has had an increase in walkouts, no-shows, cancellations, and patient complaints all focused on the amount time spent in the waiting room.
- A large pediatric practice has been experiencing an unacceptably high rate of requests for laboratory tests that ultimately do not get filled, creating frustration among both the practice staff and the patients, and potentially increasing risk to the patients.
- An ophthalmology practice wants to add an additional physician due to increasing volumes and appointment wait times, but does not have the facility space to accommodate another physician or more patients.
- For a dental practice, the cost of performing implants appears to be outpacing the price the dentists can charge in their local market.

Problem Statement. The problem statement hones in a bit more with regard to the granularity of the problem(s). It is, in a sense, a worded statement of the problem given to the interviewer by upper management. Done properly, the reader will be able to "feel" the pain of the defect, error, shortcoming, or issue being described and will gain a better understanding of the impact to the organization. And while refraining again from a lot of technical jargon, it should be specific and contain quantifiable metrics, such as time, cost, risk, etc.

One of the key components of the problem statement is that it defines the difference between where the business wants to be and where it is now, or the "gap." Gap analysis, as discussed prior, is a key concept in process improvement as it allows us to focus on the difference between current state and future state, avoiding the type of overwhelming feelings that team members tend to get when looking at the prospect of reengineering a process. Gap analysis puts the issue into perspective in such a way as to enable a higher degree of efficiency in fixing the problem.

The following are examples of problem statements:

▪ During CY 2008, approximately 2% of lab requests went unfulfilled due to no specimen collected, wrong specimen collected, specimen quantity not sufficient, and paperwork getting lost. This causes rework (the need to repeat the process), which translates into unnecessary expense; patient complaints, with a subsequent reduction in patient satisfaction; and the possibility of negatively affecting diagnoses, treatment, and the quality of care delivered. In order to ensure proper patient safety and improve efficiency, our goal is reduce this problem to under 0.1% by September 2009.

▪ Between 2007 and 2008, the number of patients walking out before their appointment nearly doubled to almost 8%. This creates an excess-capacity situation that results in increased expenses to the providers and reduced revenue through empty exam rooms. We have also noticed an increase in the number of new patients that either cancel or no-show their follow-up appointment without rescheduling. This has resulted in a 3% reduction in overall patient revenue and an increase in patient complaints with such statements as we are not competent in managing our practice. Since several of our payers also conduct patient satisfaction studies, we are concerned this may affect our position within certain PPO panels. Our goal is to reduce wait time to no more than 30 minutes, patient cycle time to no more than 60 minutes, and completely eliminate the number of walk-outs due to waiting time to zero and to complete this by July of 2009.

▪ Over the past two years, our average A/R days have increased to 51, which is 9 days over the industry average of 42. This translates to a loss in cash flow of $7200 per day creating a need to acquire short-term credit against our receivables. Within six months, our goal is to have average A/R to at least the industry average of 42 days.

Project Scope. The project scope looks at the business case and problem statement and considers the depth and the breadth of the project at hand. It details the boundaries of the project, including the start and stop points. The latter point cannot be overemphasized. At some point, you are going to have to close the project; if you don't, then after the final phases are complete, everything that even resembles the project components will begin to "creep" into the project, making it impossible to ever quantify the final outcome of your efforts. This is called "project creep," and while it is important to identify it, it can often be avoided by having a good project scope.

Following are examples of project scope statements:

- The project will be limited to examination of in-office techniques for implant surgery for efficiency. It will also involve conducting a competitive analysis of prices for other dentists along with development of a system to competitively shop for supplies and insurance. The project will begin on 9/1/09 and conclude on 12/1/09.

- In order to accommodate additional patients and providers, it is apparent that we need to find another location that will accommodate more physicians and an increase in patient visits, with adequate parking, safety, and comfort. Our search will be limited to a two-mile radius of zip code 33763 and must be completed by 1/1/2010.

- In order to reduce the number of wrong chart-pulls to zero, we will create an A3 team to create a series of solutions to be tested and presented to the administration. The team will commence on June 1 and conclude on July 1 with final presentation and solution implantation complete by July 15.

Project Goals. This step is often completed earlier in the define process but without a full understanding of the problem and the scope; therefore, it often needs to be amended and/or rewritten. Waiting until after the scope has been complete provides a better perspective on what is doable and what is not. For example, if you were to set a goal of reducing A/R to 30 days within three months and realized that you are hamstrung by your incoming EMR system until August, you would have to adjust the goal to possibly three months after stabilization has been achieved.

The project goals statement quantifies what it is you are trying to achieve and gets more granular about the measurement process. It lists target goals and objectives, including dates, times, and quantifiable results. It is still brief; and while it may require more technical language to describe some of the measurement systems and techniques, it should still be readable by those who will be required to approve the project. Remember, goals don't contain solutions or root causes. If these are included here, it is for one of two reasons: either you are making assumptions without data, which creates a bias that will likely influence the project in the wrong direction producing wrong results; or it is because you already know the root cause and solution, in which case, there wouldn't be any need to proceed. The former is often a problem we find when involving upper level management in this step because through either anecdotal experience or ego (or both), they seem to believe that they already know what needs to be done. Often, the language in the prior documents and the goals statement may cross, creating a bit of redundancy, but that is not always a bad thing as the wording is often couched differently increasing the level of understanding across the spectrum of experiences representing the people involved.

The following are examples of project goal statements:

- By February 2009, our practice will reduce the time it takes for new patients to complete registration forms from 22 minutes to 10 minutes without increasing costs.
- By the end of the year, 90% of patients will complete their entire visit within 60 minutes without a reduction in quality of care.
- By January 30, we will find a new physical plant within one mile of a residential area that will be able to accommodate five providers and three nurse practitioners.
- We will reduce the number of denials due to National Correct Coding Initiative (NCCI) edit policy by 50% by the end of the first quarter.

Realistic and Achievable Milestones.   Milestones are necessary to maintain an internal accounting of work effort as well as creating a sense of credibility to upper management. Realistic milestones reflect a basic level of experience by the team, and it is often the responsibility of the team leader to cull the timetable to ensure the project stays as close to schedule as possible. Achievable milestones are different in that they relate to the final outcome rather than time components within the project itself. There is a debate about just how important it is that the concept of achievability is defined up front. Some say that it is impossible to determine in advance exactly what goals can be achieved, while others opine that even a failed hypothesis is better than underestimating the outcomes.

Roles and Responsibilities.   While my friend and co-author, Owen Dahl, did a bang-up job in his chapter on Team Building, it is worth revisiting the roles and responsibilities of the process improvement team. Contained within the charter (remember, we are still inside that tool), this component defines who is responsible for what during the project. Even though the full team is often more diverse, the basic four roles are:

- The Project Champion is the person who wants the project done and is in a position to make it happen.
- The Facilitator is responsible for keeping the team on focus and, not being a member of the team, abstains from rendering opinions or ideas.
- The Team Leader is the boss, if you will, of the team. His or her job is to enforce rules and responsibilities and stick to the agenda.
- The Team Members can be as homogeneous or heterogeneous as needed based on the project itself. For example, more complex projects that cross disciplines, departments,

or technologies, such as EMR selection and implementation, would require a more cross-functional team, which would likely involve a greater degree of heterogeneity within the team member makeup. Less complex projects, such as reducing denials due to insurance verification errors, would likely involve a more focused team of similar skill sets.

There is one other category that, while a subset of the Team Members, is important enough to be recognized here. This is the Process Owner, who is the resident expert on the process being examined. Contrary to what many administrators may believe, process owners are likely the most important of all team participants. If you are conducting a study on check-in efficiency, it is imperative that the people who actually perform the check-in task are present. If you are trying to reduce the turnaround time for a stress test, it is imperative to have the staff members who transport the patients, prepare the equipment, and process the patients as participants on the team.

In any (and every) case, each team member should have a written responsibility and should sign off that he or she has read and accepted that responsibility.

Laboratory personnel would be important to include if you were looking to develop a throughput model to monitor requisitions. The administrator would likely be the champion and lend support while monitoring progress. The phlebotomist might be the intermediary between the clinicians and the lab to develop policies to validate and verify compliance. The facilitator would ensure that there weren't any political or personality issues that might kill or cripple the project. A consultant might be called in to lend expertise in areas of data and statistical analyses. Perhaps someone from the practice's practice management system (PMS) vendor would assist with training or even customizing certain aspects of the program to assist with changes to the practice's process.

In the design and development of a project, we often forget about the cost of poor quality. Granted, we try to estimate the cost of high quality—good staff, quality equipment, proper training, etc. But how often do we try to assess the cost of the opposite side of that coin—issues like rework (doing something over that someone has already done once) or lost claims and patient records; unhappy patients; unhappy payers; unhappy staff (which sometimes leads to Qui Tam incidents); reduced cash flow; and maybe the worst of all, the potential for civil and legal problems in the practice?

The Define Toolbox

In order to complete the Define phase of DMAIC, it requires the use of certain tools, all of which are discussed in greater detail in Chapter 5.

Define Checklist

- Is the problem clear and are there data to support the problem statement?
- Are the goals clear and realistic?
- Is the problem linked to definable costs of poor quality?
- Has the benefit been estimated?
- Are the customers and what their needs are known?
- Are the project focused and the scope clear?
- Is there a team in place and ready to go?
- Is there buy-in and approval by the key management?

Measure

*When you can measure what you are talking about and
express it in numbers, you know something about it.*
—LORD WILLIAM THOMSON KELVIN

The primary goal of the Measure phase is to pinpoint the location or source of a problem as precisely as possible by building a factual understanding of existing process conditions. That knowledge helps you narrow the range of potential causes requiring investigation in the Analyze phase that follows. An important part of the Measure phase is to establish a set of baseline measurements that help define the process and the capability level. For example, how many patients a day can the practice handle and what is the industry standard? We might want to establish a current state measurement of the number of minutes it takes to get a patient through a visit cycle and maybe the ratio of FTEs-to-provider in order to compare against some other national or regional benchmark. In any case, the old adage "If you can't measure it, you can't manage it" is so very important here.

Steps in the Measure Phase

The first step in the Measure phase is to get to the understanding of process behavior. Some of this will be (or will already have been) accomplished through the use of process mapping. The visualization of the process is the first step toward understanding its behavior. The second is to determine what needs to be measured.

For example, if our project focuses on reducing (or understanding) A/R, we need to determine what data would be important to our understanding of the issue. Some practices use charges for A/R but since revenue models and charges models are basically disconnected, we will only be measuring charge A/R, which may or may not be important to the goals of the project. Maybe we estimate revenue and use that to measure our average A/R days, but since it is just about impossible to determine what to expect in payment from insurers in one out of every four claim lines, we would need to understand the range of error expected in using that type of metric. We might just use a 12-month rolling average of daily collections against average daily charges.

What becomes important is actually our next step, which is determining the methods used to measure the data quality. So often I see practices using some external source for benchmarks yet nowhere in the data are there indications of sample error, practice type, location, etc. For example, let's say that we are looking for some benchmark of the ratio of FTE staff per provider. How do we know what the relative profitability is of the practices that responded to the survey from which the data are obtained? Are they efficient? Do they have some kind of over- or under-capacity issue? How long does it take a new patient to get in to see the doctor? How many nonphysician practitioners, if any, were included in the database? You will do what you have to do in order to establish these benchmarks but establishing some policy to measure data quality early on may likely save you the problem of having to start over later.

One way to ensure continuity and consistency in this phase is to have a written data collection plan. There are many examples of formal and informal written data collection plans on the Internet, but most conform to the following questions:

- What do you need to know?
- What types of data will provide you with the information that you need?
- What types of data are already available to you (existing archival sources and other artifacts)?
- From where will the data originate?
- Who will be responsible for the data collection?
- Who will be responsible to validate accuracy?
- Will you need outside assistance?
- When (by what date) will the data be required in order to keep with the time line?

Often, we need to conduct a probe analysis (an initial small study) to help us determine such important things like sample size. You might be surprised to find that, irrespective of what it is you are trying to measure, someone may have already done a study similar to the one you are planning. Access to these data can help you to estimate parameters, such as variability, which are important for size determinations. Existing studies will often save you a bunch of time and money and help to move the project along.

One set of benchmarks that the practice will want to establish are internal, such as number of patients required to break even, cost per RVU, number of patients per provider per day, or visit capacity levels. Depending on what is being measured, external benchmarks are far less important than the internal ones; and with internal benchmarks, at least you can have more control over and a better understanding of the accuracy and validity of the results.

Data collection can sometimes seem a bit overwhelming, especially to folks who may not be used to working with large amounts of information. Even though much of what you are going to do later is dependent upon the measurement phase, remember to keep it as simple as possible. Ensure that the methods for measuring are focused on data that are meaningful to the project. I work with a lot of CPAs who are involved with medical practices. If you heard me talking about cost accounting and one of them talking about cost accounting, you might think that there were two completely different topics being discussed. I have often seen the voluminous cost accounting reports that have been commissioned by the practice and performed by a competent CPA sit on the shelf and collect dust; not because the information is incorrect but because it is not what the practice needed in order to make improvement or understand its processes. From a more Lean perspective, what we measure should be directly attributable to a specific goal, and having too much information is just as spurious as having too little. When process participants collect meaningless data for management purposes, it undermines the support and trust of data collection systems because no positive results can be seen coming from the effort.

The Measure Toolbox

As mentioned above, each phase has its own set of tools, and the following are some that we often find as a part of the measure phase:

- Value Stream Mapping (VSM)
- Data and Statistics
- Sampling
- Prioritization Matrices
- Process Cycle Efficiency
- Pareto Charts
- Control Charts
- Run Charts

What Should You Measure?

In a well-written data collection plan, this will be covered in detail. First, you need to identify the measurable data within the process. This is a key component of VSM; refer back to

Chapter 5, and review what goes into the data box for each step in the process map. It may be earnings before interest and tax, cycle time, denial rate, A/R, turnover, or any number of other quantifiable metrics. As mentioned, you need to identify the source of the data, such as the PMS, a P&L statement, or a tax return. Sometimes, you need data that initially seems nonquantifiable, such as HR records. But remember, if it can't be quantified (or measured), it is unlikely that you can set a specific goal, and there may not be a good candidate for this type of process improvement model. Sometimes the source of the data will be an outside vendor, such as a billing service, or you may require assistance from an existing vendor, such as help with creating certain reports from your PMS.

In establishing a baseline analysis, you should consider using control charts, time series analyses, statistical measurements, etc. It is important to understand the ranges of significance in many of the studies that you will conduct. And while many of the types of statistical tests that are both available and valuable are outside the scope of this book, it would behoove every reader to spend some time brushing up on their understanding of basic statistics. There are lots of good books, such as *Statistics for Dummies*, available for little cost. You can also go to the author's Web site at www.frankcohen.com and view free webinars on statistics for healthcare professionals. In any case, irrespective of what you collect, it is important to be able to define the difference between what is necessary and what is nice to know. Much of your direction will occur in the next phase (Analyze) as a result of what you measure here; so to the best of your ability, try to focus on the bigger picture.

In an A/R project, you would want to obtain such data as charges, collections, aging reports, write-off projections, bad debt, patient responsibility, etc. If you are looking at the billing cycle, you might want to know how long it takes from checkout until the claim gets filed, how many claims are denied as a percent of claim lines, or even what percent of denied claims are reversed on appeal and why. Certainly, knowing the total time from claim submission to final adjudication would be a very important measurement here. In a patient throughput cycle analysis, you would likely want to measure the time for each and all of the steps in the cycle, including check-in time, wait time, visit time, etc.

If you are working on a coding improvement project, you might want to measure relative risk through benchmarking the practice's ratios against some control group, like Medicare or UHC data. You might want to compare the relative utilization of procedure codes and/or modifiers against the national or state benchmarks for physicians in similar specialties. It may be as simple as measuring the rate of audit reversals both before and after training. Perhaps you are considering getting an EMR system and want to set up a process in advance to control implementation. For sure, you would want to benchmark work RVUs per provider at least six months prior to the changeover, during the implementation, and for several months afterward to assess the loss of productivity during the implementation phase and see if you are able to return to where you were before the conversion began.

A couple of tools that work very well together in this phase are the CTQ tree and the key process indicator (KPI) diagram. We discussed these in detail in the Chapter 5, but due to their importance, they bear a bit of repeat here. Let's take an example of a CTQ that deals with wait-time issues.

The CTQ tree in Figure 1 examines the drivers behind reducing wait time to a goal of, say, 25 minutes. For example, in order to reduce wait time, you would need an efficient intake procedure. And in order to do that, you would need to have the chart available and payer information validated quickly. The KPI diagram (Figure 2) would then detail what measurements would be needed in order to satisfy each of the drivers.

In our example above, the CTQ drivers were available charts and quick insurance verification. Here, the KPIs would be the percent of events in which the chart was not available and the number of times that payer verification took longer than five minutes. The data needed for the former would be total patient encounters and ratio of missing charts;

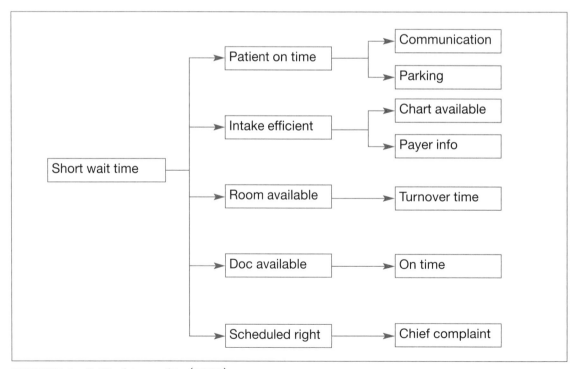

FIGURE 1. Critical-to-quality (CTQ) tree.

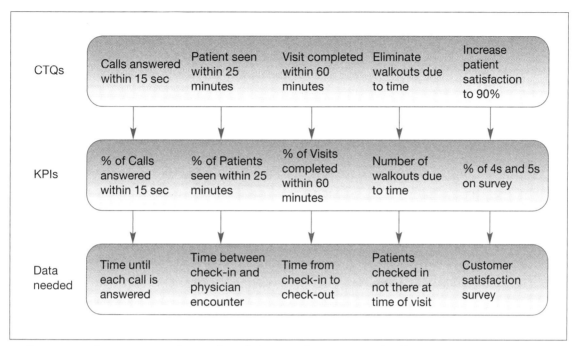

FIGURE 2. A key process indicator (KPI) diagram for a variety of different CTQ items.

and for payer verification, data needed would include total patient encounters and time to verification for each.

Once again, the data collection plan should be a guide to assist you along the way. One of the questions that should be incorporated is: Does the practice even have the capability to collect the data? Let's say that you are going to conduct a denial analysis; and in addition to measuring the volume of claims that are denied as a percent of the claims submitted (say, by week), you also want to analyze the reason codes given for the denial by payer. In order to do this, you would either need to have a PMS that could extract this from the 835 form or ERA (assuming you are submitting electronically) or from the EOB if you are submitting manually (by mail). Many PMSs are not capable of doing this so you would have to contract with an outside company, such as NHXS (nhxs.com), to get the data to conduct the analysis.

Once again, the types of data and statistics you will be reviewing is outside the scope of this book but that does not change the reality of the need. It would be nice to understand the difference between types of variables, such as continuous and discreet. It is important to have a basic understanding of distribution families in order to determine whether using the mean or the median would be the most accuracy estimate of central tendency. Knowing the variability of the data is critical for understanding sampling error as is the direction and magnitude of relationships, such as payer mix and revenue.

Descriptive Statistics: Check-in to Exam Room

Variable	Mean	StDev	Variance	Median	Range	IQR	Mode
Clock-in to Exam Room	36.15	15.47	239.37	32.00	73.00	23.75	23, 24, 27

FIGURE 3. **Time (in minutes) from check-in to exam room. IQR, interquartile range; StDev, standard deviation.**

One very salient point deals with how data are going to be presented, and it is always (note the word "always") better to include graphs along with your table. In data-intense situations, a picture is worth at least a thousand cells. Let's take a look at some examples of the type of data you might want to collect and the different ways to present them.

In a study of patient visit cycle time, you examine the time from check-in to exam room. The data table might be simple, like the one shown in Figure 3.

Figure 3 shows that the mean is higher than the median, indicating that the data might be right-skewed and that the median may be a better measurement. It also reports the variability as well as the mode—which number(s) appeared the most.

Figure 4 is a more detailed representation of the data in a graphic format, and it shows a story that the table couldn't: not only are the data not normally distributed, but the histogram shows a bimodal state. That is, there are two peaks instead of one.

As you gain experience in data collection and analysis, you will see that this indicates there are actually two separate states rather than just one. In this case, the distribution on the left is for established patients while the distribution on the right is for new patients. This would indicate the need to conduct two studies: one on the time for new patients and one on the time for established patients. You can also see the positional characteristics of the mean and the median as well the variability and the range of statistical significance, called the confidence interval (CI).

While some of you may not want (or need) this much information, the idea is to have the ability to collect as much as you need to make this phase meaningful and valuable.

In one practice, there was a concern that one of the providers spent a significantly longer amount of time with patients (both new and established) than the other two providers. In fact, initial studies did show that the average time for that physician was, in fact, significantly longer. Figure 5 is a boxplot of time statistics for each of the physicians broken down by new and established patients.

One again, the picture represented here speaks volumes to those assumptions. Here, we see that each of the three physicians averaged about the same time for both new and

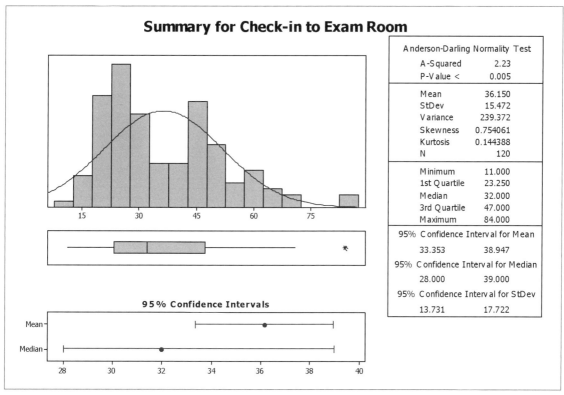

FIGURE 4. Summary for check-in to exam room. StDev, standard deviation.

established patients, indicating that there isn't, in fact, any differences. Why, then, did the initial time study show that the average for Physician 1 was so much higher? The answer, it turned out, is that the physician in question saw a lot more new patients, and since the overall time for new patients was greater, his overall time was also more than that of his co-workers.

Figure 6 gives an example of a physician productivity study. Profitability is a ratio of revenue over expense, so to measure the profitability of a physician, you need to know his or her total collections and total expenses. It's pretty simple, actually. Productivity, however, is a measurement of the relationship between each physician's revenue as a percent of total revenue and his or her expenses as a percent of total expenses. The goal is to have a ratio of 1; what the physician contributes to the practice as a percent of total is the same as what he or she consumes as a percent of the total.

Here, we can see that the expense productivity values for the doctors are all over the board.

Perhaps what is more telling is that the median productivity is 0.97, below what would be expected from a practice reporting average productivity.

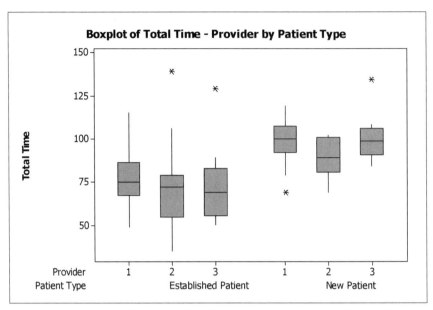

FIGURE 5. Boxplot of time statistics for each of the physicians broken down by new and established patients. The asterisks represent outliers.

Provider ID	Specialty	Percent Charges	Percent Revenue	Percent RVU	Percent Work RVU	Percent Expense	RVU Productivity Ratio	Expense Productivity Ratio
13	IM	4.96%	6.64%	5.05%	4.46%	3.91%	1.31	1.70
66	GE	6.56%	6.81%	6.43%	7.03%	9.44%	1.06	0.72
71	PM	7.45%	6.19%	6.79%	5.53%	5.84%	0.91	1.06
95	GE	7.32%	7.04%	8.19%	10.10%	9.46%	0.86	0.74
1025	RH	2.54%	3.44%	3.13%	4.03%	4.19%	1.10	0.82
1056	PM	6.75%	5.03%	7.59%	8.92%	5.50%	0.66	0.91
120	EN	2.73%	2.70%	3.03%	2.88%	2.04%	0.89	1.33
1249	IM	3.43%	4.38%	4.46%	5.03%	3.53%	0.98	1.24
1262	IM	6.17%	6.57%	6.94%	5.69%	4.33%	0.95	1.52
136	GE	9.80%	9.78%	8.47%	7.33%	10.18%	1.15	0.96
1633	IM	2.91%	3.47%	3.76%	5.29%	3.20%	0.92	1.08
170	GE	9.14%	8.70%	7.79%	6.23%	10.10%	1.12	0.86
794	GR	2.10%	2.08%	2.92%	3.94%	2.92%	0.71	0.71
8	RH	7.80%	8.92%	6.63%	5.66%	5.21%	1.34	1.71
519	UR	13.04%	10.89%	12.86%	10.39%	11.13%	0.85	0.98
873	GS	7.30%	7.38%	5.95%	7.50%	9.04%	1.24	0.82
Lower Range		2.10%	2.08%	2.92%	2.88%	2.04%	0.66	0.71
Lower Quartile		3.30%	4.15%	4.29%	4.89%	3.81%	0.88	0.82
Mean		6.25%	6.25%	6.25%	6.25%	6.25%	1.00	1.07
Median		6.65%	6.60%	6.53%	5.68%	5.36%	0.96	0.97
Upper Quartile		7.54%	7.71%	7.64%	7.37%	9.45%	1.13	1.26
Upper Range		13.04%	10.89%	12.86%	10.39%	11.13%	1.34	1.71
Standard Deviation		2.93%	2.50%	2.49%	2.10%	2.99%	0.19	0.32

FIGURE 6. Physician productivity study.

Provider ID	Specialty	E/M Time	Non-E/M Time	Total Time
8	RH	489	1,854	2,344
13	IM	1,278	741	2,020
66	GE	2,283	1,403	3,686
71	PM	1,021	1,339	2,360
95	GE	4,030	1,180	5,211
120	EN	1,322	4	1,327
136	GE	811	2,188	2,999
170	GE	827	1,893	2,720
519	UR	1,006	2,511	3,517
794	GR	2,040	-	2,040
873	GS	458	2,320	2,779
1025	RH	1,903	7	1,911
1056	PM	3,531	742	4,273
1249	IM	2,337	48	2,386
1262	IM	2,475	127	2,603
1633	IM	2,525	-	2,525
		28,336	16,357	44,701
Lower Range		458	-	1,327
Lower Quartile		961	38	2,268
Mean		1,771	1,022	2,794
Median		1,613	961	2,564
Upper Quartile		2,372	1,864	3,129
Upper Range		4,030	2,511	5,211
Standard Deviation		1,022	903	941

FIGURE 7. **Provider time analysis table.**

Staying on the topic of physicians, if this were a compliance improvement project, you might want to take a look at the number of hours assessed for each physician under the Harvard/Relative Value Scale Update Committee (RUC) time study. This is the study that assigns time values to a variety of procedures and services and is used to establish the Work and Practice Expense RVU values. The Office of Inspector General is known to be suspicious of providers that report in excess of 5000 assessed hours, which is 2.5 times the stated fair market value benchmark of 2000 hours. To measure this, you multiply the number of minutes for each procedure times the number of times the procedure was performed, total the products, and then divide by 60 to get hours. Do this for each provider and look at the number of total hours. Note in the example shown in Figure 7 that provider 95 reports a total assessed time of 5211 hours—211 hours in excess of the presumed audit threshold.

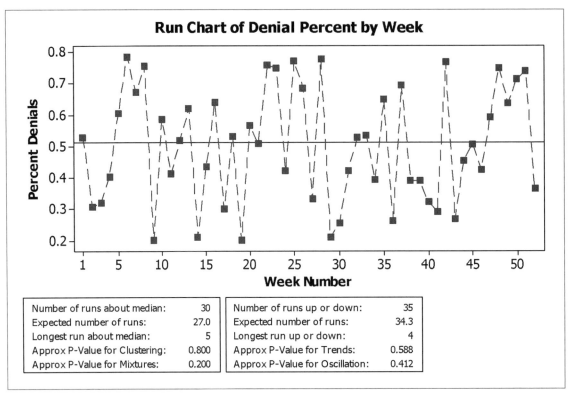

FIGURE 8. Run chart of denial rates per week.

Many practices engage in coding improvement projects. Even those that focus on A/R and cash flow involve a review and/or analysis of denials. Two important metrics are the number of claim lines denied as a percent of total claim lines and the reason codes for those denials. Run charts and Pareto graphs are great ways to measure these data.

Figure 8 provides a great visualization of the patterns, characteristics, central tendency, and variability of denials from week to week. Some statistics packages will also create a test for clustering, trends, and oscillation.

The Pareto chart shown in Figure 9 is a great way to visualize the impact that each reason code has on the reported denials. Note how it organizes the reason codes into buckets such that it is easy to see that reason codes 27 and 38 make up more than 80% of all reason codes. This is a great way to become "underwhelmed" in what often feels like an overwhelming project.

If you wanted to get even more granular, you could break down reason codes by category, such as is illustrated in Figure 10. In this graph, we can see, for example, that reason code 38 is pretty much exclusive to E/M codes.

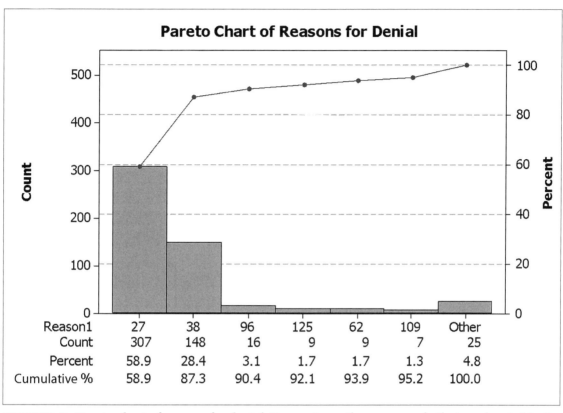

Pareto Chart of Reasons for Denial

Reason1	27	38	96	125	62	109	Other
Count	307	148	16	9	9	7	25
Percent	58.9	28.4	3.1	1.7	1.7	1.3	4.8
Cumulative %	58.9	87.3	90.4	92.1	93.9	95.2	100.0

FIGURE 9. Pareto chart of reasons for denial. Reason1 was the reason code that was located in the first position of the denial.

One very important area of process improvement and management is the acquisition and implementation of EMR systems. Knowing whether the expense incurred (approximately $25,000 per physicians as of this writing) resulted in any kind of return on investment is critically important, and being able to track progress or decomposition of the productivity is absolutely essential in order to determine whether stability has been achieved. As shown in Figure 11, we measured denials due to medical necessity six months prior to implementation and six months after implementation was complete. In this figure, the lower control limit (LCL) represents the lower end of the acceptable range calculated by the model. More likely, however, when we are looking to minimize an event, we would enter the LCL as zero, since the goal would be to have no denials due to medical necessity. The upper control limit (UCL) calculates the upper limit such that any points that appear above it should be reviewed to determine the cause. The X represents the actual average percent of denials across the spectrum of data.

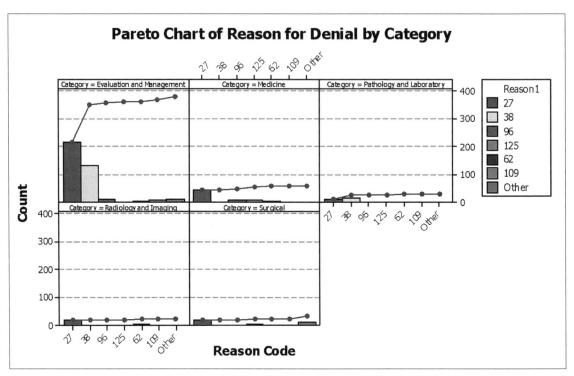

FIGURE 10. Pareto chart of reasons for denial by category.

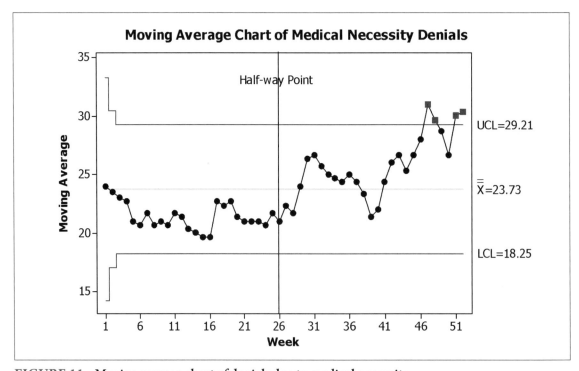

FIGURE 11. Moving average chart of denials due to medical necessity.

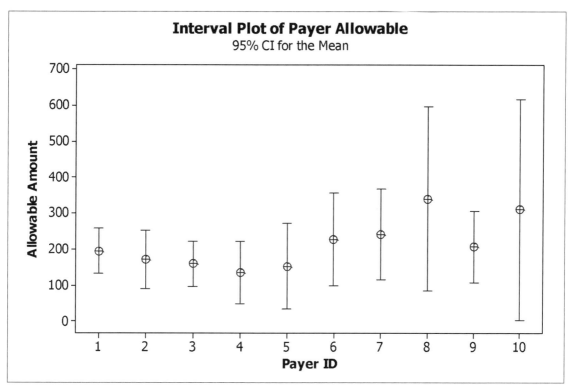

FIGURE 12. Interval plot of payments from different payers (95% CI for the mean).

Note here the trend of increasing denials due to medical necessity *after* final implementation and the system was up and running. This may indicate any number of issues, including possible over coding by physicians due to the ease of increasing documentation.

Understanding payer behavior is very important when it comes to conducting a revenue cycle analysis. As shown in Figure 12, we measured the average reimbursement against the practice's usual and customary fee, along with the 95% confidence intervals in order to get a better idea as to what the entire population of collections looks like.

Note here how some payers, such as payers 8 and 10, have a wider range of appropriate reimbursement than, say, payer 1 or 3.

Sometimes, we use control charts in the measurement phase to get an idea as to the process capability. In the example shown in Figure 13, we looked at patient satisfaction data by week for a one-year period in order to establish a baseline measurement as well as to get an idea as to what the practice was capable of regarding overall patient satisfaction scores. In this chart, any point above the UCL would indicate that something occurred during that period that caused the process to be "out of control." The same rule would apply here for data points below the LCL. As with most of the other charts represented in

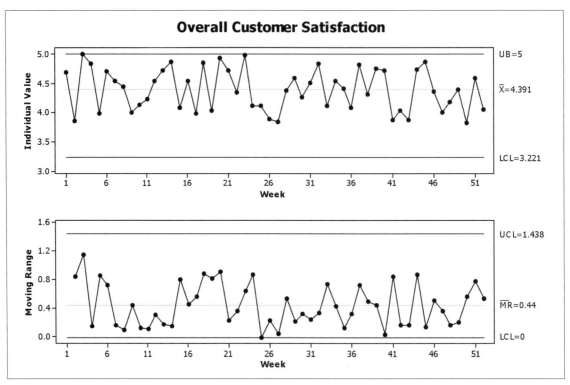

FIGURE 13. Overall customer satisfaction. The moving range (MR) plots the difference between the data points.

this chapter, X, either with or without a bar above it, represents the mathematical average for the data represented in the chart.

The benefit here is it gives us the ability to look at gap analysis when setting goals. For example, we may be happy with the average score of 4.391 (on a scale of 5) but we want to reduce the variability so that three standard deviations remain within a range of 4.0 to 4.9.

MSA Drilldown. Measurement system analysis (MSA) drilldown is a structured approach to checking the quality of your data. Its principle is that you should not be using data if you do not know where the data came from, and an MSA drilldown helps to challenge the "pedigree" of the data. A "tree" diagram may be the best way to structure the results.

Take a look at the tree diagram in Figure 14 for examining the characteristics for measuring the time from check-in to exam room.

In some ways, this is similar to the CTQ tree. For example, in order to measure time from check-in to exam room, we need to define what defines both the start and the stop time. Let's say we agree that the measurement begins when the patient checks in at the front desk.

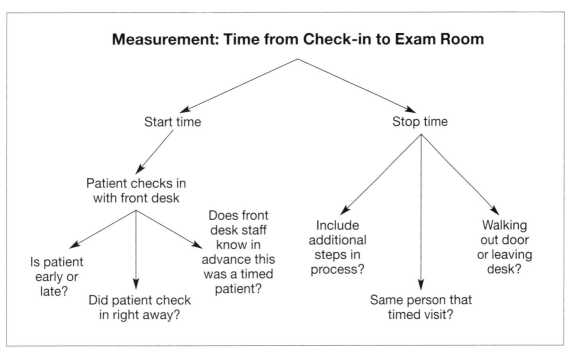

FIGURE 14. **Measurement: time from check-in to exam room.**

What if the patient is late or early? Do we count from the time the patient arrives or the actual scheduled time of the appointment? Did the timing start when it was supposed to—did the staff know that this was a timed patient? Did the patient check in right away or did he or she just come in and sit down in the waiting room? Maybe the patient signed in at the desk but no one was there. Do we start the clock when the patient arrived (we don't know how long he or she has been waiting) or when the check-in procedure begins? The same holds true for when to stop.

Unless these issues are addressed in the front end of the measurement phase, you open yourself up to both inaccurate and inconsistent data; and by now, you know the consequences of that. Decisions made based on bad data are bad decisions.

Sample Size. The final comment I want to make concerning the measure phase is that of sample size. Depending on the level of criticality of your project, sample size may play a very important role. Too large a sample wastes time and money, while too small a sample may not give enough information to be of value.

Here's a great (and very common) example. A Recovery Audit Contractor (RAC) auditor will come in to a practice and request 10 charts. Let's say the auditor pulls 10 visits reporting a 99214. The audit concludes that three of these should have been a 99213. Let's say that the difference in reimbursement between a 99214 and a 99213 is $32, and let's also say that the practice reported a total of 1500 code 99214s. In an extrapolation recovery, the RAC will likely take the 30% rate of disagreement and multiply it times the universe of 99214 codes reported (1500,) and conclude that 30% of them (450) should have been reported as a 99213. Multiply the $32 times the 450, and the repayment demand is $14,400.

Here's the $14,400 question: what is 3 divided by 10? Seems pretty simple, right? It's 30%; but is it really? This is a case of inferential statistics—using the results of a small sample to infer a conclusion to a population; and the fact is, in any sample, there is going to be error. How much error is critical in this type of audit. If we were to conduct a one-proportion test for 3 events in 10 trials, we would see that the true range of 3 divided by 10 is somewhere between 6.7% and 65.2%. Maybe you could negotiate toward the bottom of this 95% CI, say a 10% discrepancy rather than a 30% discrepancy. This could reduce the repayment demand from $14,400 to $4800. How about if the auditor pulled 100 charts and found 30 in disagreement? It's still not 30%; it's somewhere between 21.2% and 40%.

As you can see, the larger the sample size the smaller the confidence interval. And while it isn't always a good idea to increase sample size (what if they find 40 disagreements in 100 charts rather than 30?), it is always important to understand the significance of sample size and sample selection.

In sample size selection, there are several parameters that are normally considered; and while it can be a complex area, there are some ways to simplify it. Following are some tips and examples that may help. The two parameters that we tend to control are the confidence interval and the sensitivity of the results. The CI is a value that allows us to infer the relative accuracy of our sample compared with the total population. For example, when a poll is conducted to project the winner of the presidential election, it is necessary to survey only around 2000 people to infer the results to the entire voting population plus or minus 3%. With a 95% CI, this means that we could be 95% sure that if we were able to collect the response from every possible respondent, the actual ratio would be somewhere within that 6% total range. This is, however, dependent on the validity of the randomness of the sample, which will be discussed shortly.

Regarding CIs, the higher the CI, the greater the range and the more applicable to situations that require greater criticality. For example, for an internal review, you may be happy with a 90% CI. For an external audit, it may be 95%. If there is litigation involved, 99% may be a more realistic target. For some clinical studies, 99.9% is required. In order to use the upcoming formula, the CI needs to be converted to a z-score, something we can't discuss here but the values are as follows:

90.0% = 1.645
95.0% = 1.96
99.0% = 2.58
99.9% = 3.30

The next question deals with the sensitivity (or acceptable error) for our measurements. The formula is $n = (Z * S)^2/h$, which reads as follows: the number of samples we need (n) is equal to the z-score for the confidence interval (Z) times the estimated standard deviation (S) squared divided by the sensitivity of our measurement (h). Again, for critical experiments, the formula is more complex than presented here, but for many internal analyses, this formula will prove to be sufficient. For example, let's say that you want to study average wait time from check-in to exam room, and you want to be 95% confident that the true average for all patients is within plus or minus 5 minutes of your results. In a prior study, you learned that the average wait time was 44.15 minutes with a standard deviation of 12.5 minutes.

Here, Z = 1.96 (95% CI), S = 12.5 minutes, and h = 5 minutes (sensitivity or noise from normal variability). The formula would then be 1.96 times 12.5 squared (600.25) divided by 5, and result in n = 120. This means that you would need a sample size of around 120 to have a statistically significant result.

The final consideration is the concept of randomness. In a truly random sample, every single member of the population has to have an exactly equal chance of being selected. A complete discussion of random sampling techniques is beyond the scope of this book, however, that does not diminish its importance. It would behoove the reader to do a bit of background reading on sample size selection but just remember, any time one sample has a greater chance of being included than another, it introduces bias into the equation.

Analyze

> *The art of discovering the causes of phenomena, or true*
> *hypothesis, is like the art of deciphering, in which an*
> *ingenious conjecture greatly shortens the road.*
> —Gottfried Wilhelm Leibniz

The analysis phase is designed to identify what factors define a "gold standard" for a product or service and the reason for the problems found within the project. It is during this step that you identify the gap between where you are and where you need to be and just what specific issues are holding you back.

The steps in the analyze phase are as follows:

1. Analyze the process.
2. Develop theories and ideas about root causes.
3. Verify the root causes.
4. Get an understanding of the cause-and-effect relationship.
5. Verify all assumptions with the team.

And the following are some of the major tools that will be needed:

1. Process Mapping
2. VSM
3. Data Analysis
4. Brainstorming, Fishbone diagram
5. Cause and Effect, Failure Mode Effect Analysis

First, let's look at the steps one, well, step at a time.

Analyzing the Process

The first step is to analyze the process. By this time, you have already created the process map, which gives you a visual understanding of the flow of patients, products, and/or services from start to finish. Figure 15 is a map of a fee schedule development and maintenance process.

Visualizing the process makes it much easier to understand the "how" and the "why" of what goes, on and its value cannot be understated. Analyzing the process, however, begins with an additional tool: VSM. Like process mapping, VSM has been discussed in detail in Chapter 5, and therefore we will not repeat it here, but it is worth noting again an example of what a value stream map might look like (Figure 16).

As you can see, we have used the map here to dissect and analyze a number of different metrics for each step in the process. For example, we know that 15.4% of patients are late. From an analytical perspective, to get more granular on this issue, what is it that we would want to know in order to be able to improve the efficiency (and reduce waste; in this case it is time) during the check-in step of the patient visit process? It would be to understand the "why" of that metric. We would also want to create a financial impact analysis in order to support a benefit-risk analysis for the resources that may be required for any change.

For example, let's say that the practice sees 140 patients per day. This would mean that around 22 patients per day were late. It would be a great idea to determine the total and average amount of time that is involved in this, so we would record the number of minutes

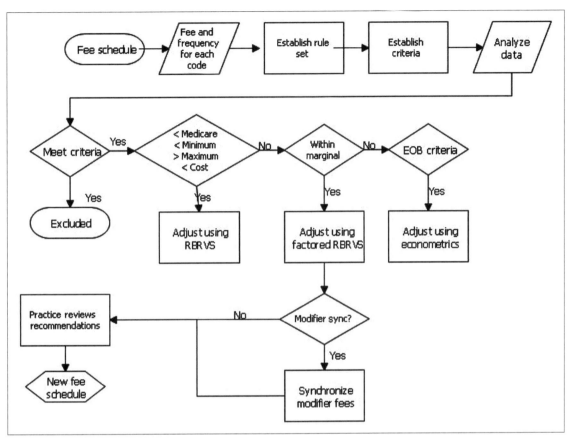

FIGURE 15. Fee schedule development and maintenance process. EOB, explanation of benefits.

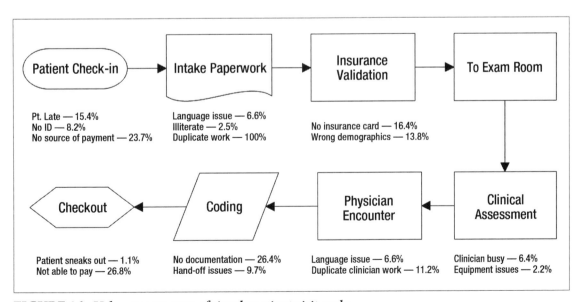

FIGURE 16. Value stream map of simple patient visit cycle.

Patient Late	Doctor Wait
7	5
23	12
14	10
26	0
31	14
7	0
23	14
7	2
31	6

FIGURE 17. **Sample of data from late patients.**

late for each patient. And if the physician had to wait for a room, we would calculate how many minutes were involved in that wasted time.

Figure 17 contains 10 random samples for patients that were late.

When we look at the data for all patients late and all doctors' wait time for one day, we see a scatter graph that looks like the one shown in Figure 18.

Note that there is very little correlation between late patients and physician wait time. This tells us that while we could predict the number of patients that will be late on any given day (and how late they might be) and how often a provider waits with an empty room for a late patient (and how long the provider will wait), we cannot accurately predict the provider wait time based on the patient late time. This is important as it helps to move us into a different direction.

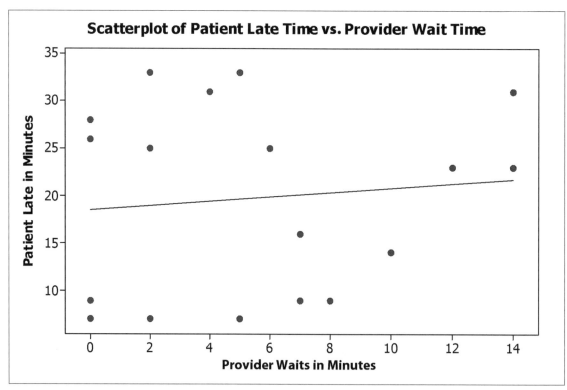

FIGURE 18. **Scatterplot of late patients vs. provider wait time.**

Nonetheless, we are able to calculate the total number of minutes associated with late patients on a given day (371), the average minutes for each late patient (16.86), the total minutes doctors spent waiting with an empty room (211), and the average wait time per late event (9.59 minutes). If we go a step further and analyze the potential costs to the practice, we begin to reach the point where our data can be translated into something quite useful.

Let's look at the number of minutes the providers spend waiting with an empty room since this can be immediately associated with a loss in revenue for the practice. In a different analysis of revenue over time, we calculated that the average revenue per hour for a provider is $261. If you multiply the $261 times 3.5 hours (the 211 minutes the provider waits with an empty room), you can estimate that late patients are costing the practice $913.50 per day, $4567 per week, $19,640 per month, and upwards of $235,683 per year.

Another way to look at this would be to estimate the number of patients seen per hour and the average revenue per visit. For example, let's say that this practice could see three patients per hour with average revenue of $90 per visit. In this case, we would multiply the 3.5 hours of wasted time by three patient visits per hour to get a total of 10.5 additional patients per day. Using this as a basis for our calculations, we end up with a loss of 2167 visits per year with a potential revenue of $195,048. Either way, the financial impact is quite large. The final task in the analysis of this step would be to understand why the patients are late, and this is easily accomplished by asking the patients (rather than assuming you know).

Imagine the power of what we have seen so far. By analyzing just this one factor (patient late time), we are able to figure out a solution that could generate hundreds of thousands of dollars a year in additional revenue without adding any additional cost (less variable expense). This truly epitomizes the concept, application, and practicality of process improvement.

Let's continue on with an example that we have touched on in the past: patient visit cycle. We have already looked at defining the problems, mapping the process, and creating benchmarks and metrics for analysis. Let's go further, and take a look at how we might analyze this type of process in order to find a way to reduce waste within the system and improve the consistency of the different steps that take place.

In this example, we are dealing with a three-physician medical practice that has seen an increase in the time patients wait to be seen and the overall time it takes for the entire visit cycle. This has resulted in an increase in walkouts, cancellations, and no-shows over the past year or so and has also been associated with a decrease in overall patient satisfaction scores. The practice administrator believes that this is likely due to one of the doctors taking significantly longer to see patients and process their charts through to check-out, creating a bottleneck for waiting patients and availability of rooms. One suggestion was to hire a physician assistant in order to pick up the backlog of patients for that physician.

For this situation, we have defined the problem: excessive wait time and patient visit cycle. Through mapping the process, we defined which metrics needed to be studied, and these were check-in time, wait-room time, exam room time, and check-out time. To do this in accordance with the prior phase, a sample size analysis was conducted, and it was determined that we should capture time-based metrics for six patients a day; three in the morning and three in the afternoon every day for a month. To ensure randomness, times were preselected, and the next patient to check-in after the designated time was selected for the study.

We started with an overall look at total time from check-in to check-out, and the findings are summarized in Figure 19.

This summary analysis, taken from the program MiniTab (MiniTab, Inc.), gives us a plethora of valuable information. For example, it helps to benchmark our current state, reporting an average visit cycle time of 82 minutes. It also shows that the data follow a normal distribution, making it easier to predict the location characteristics of other times within the model. For example, with a standard deviation of 19.5, we could estimate that, for 68% of patients, the average wait time was between 62.5 and 101.5 minutes. For 95% of patients, the total visit time was somewhere between 43 minutes and 121 minutes. We can also see a CI of 78.4 to 85.4, meaning that we are 95% confident that the true average visit cycle time for all patients is somewhere between 78.4 and 85.4 minutes.

The next step was to see if there was any significant difference among days of the week. For example, is patient visit cycle time longer on Friday than on Wednesday? Figure 20 shows what is known as an ANOVA, or analysis of variance. This measures the difference between the averages by day to determine any significant variance.

Using this method, while we are able to see that the averages for each day were different, based on our sample size, we determined that the differences were due to normal variability, or noise, and not considered significantly different. There are two ways that this can be determined. First is to look at the P value on the top line of data. If it is above 0.05, it indicates that the averages are essentially the same. The other is to look at the histogram for each day. As long as the intervals overlap, we would determine they are basically the same.

One staff person suggested that new patients seemed to consistently wait longer than established patients. As a result, we separated the data into new and existing patients and

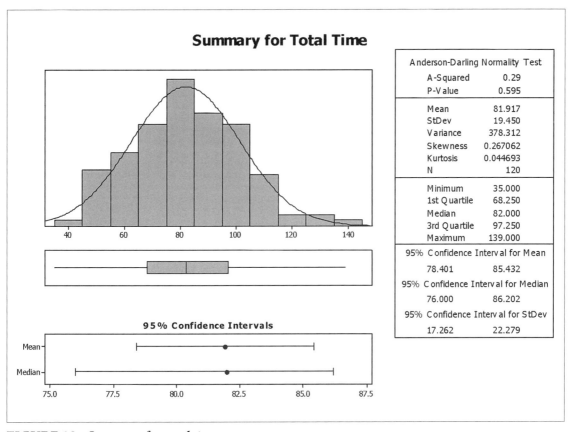

FIGURE 19. Summary for total time.

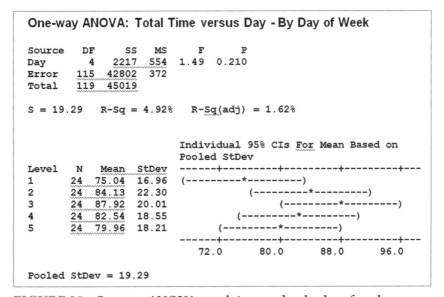

FIGURE 20. One-way ANOVA: total time vs. day, by day of week.

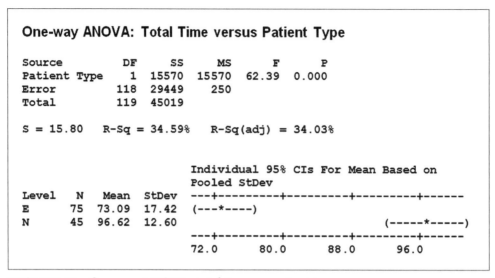

FIGURE 21. One-way ANOVA: total time vs. patient type.

conducted a significance test to see if, in fact, this was an anecdotal observation or if there was really something to it.

The analysis shown in Figure 21 indicates that, indeed, total visit cycle time was heavily influenced by the type of patient (new vs. established).

This can be observed both by the fact that the P value is below 0.05 and that the intervals in the histogram do not overlap. Here, we see that established patients average 73 minutes while new patients average almost 97 minutes—a significant difference.

The next step was to analyze the difference between the four measurement points: check-in to exam room, exam room to provider (the second waiting room), provider time, and time to check-out. To do this, we created a series of scatterplots to study the relationship for each of these factors to total time (Figure 22).

Note that of the four contributing factors, check-in to exam room and provider time had the greatest effect on total time, with check-in to exam room taking an easy first place. This is determined based on the closely associated pattern of data points on the graph.

The next step was to analyze wait time by patient type, since we had established that patient type had a significant influence over total time, and then to take a look at the time each physician spent with the patient for all patients and also by patient type.

To do this, we used what is called a box-and-whisker plot, which visualizes the average time, relative variability, and overall range of the data points (Figure 23). This graph shows a clear difference for all physicians and all visits between new and established patients. This

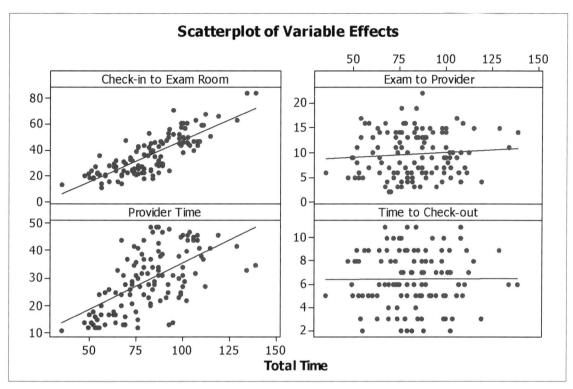

FIGURE 22. Scatterplots of check-in to exam room, exam room to provider, provider time, and time to check-out.

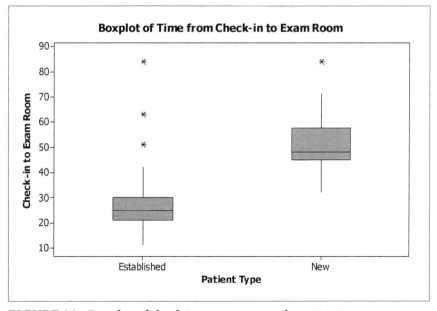

FIGURE 23. Boxplot of check-in to exam room, by patient type.

```
Two-Sample T-Test and CI

Sample    N    Mean   StDev   SE Mean
1         75   27.20  10.7        1.2
2         45   51.04  9.62        1.4


Difference = mu (1) - mu (2)
Estimate for difference:  -23.83
95% CI for difference:  (-27.58, -20.08)
T-Test of difference = 0 (vs not =):
T-Value = -12.60   P-Value = 0.000   DF = 100
```

FIGURE 24. Statistical representation of boxplot in Figure 23.

is a very common graph type for this kind of analysis, and you should commit some time to becoming comfortable with its use and interpretation.

The statistical test in Figure 24 shows that there is, in fact, a statistically significant difference between the two samples here where new patients are represented by the number 2 in the sample and established patients by the number 1. Again, it shows that P < 0.05; and in this test, if there was not a significant difference, the range for the 95% CI for difference would include zero, which it clearly does not.

When we conducted the same test to examine provider time by patient type, we saw something both interesting and unexpected: there doesn't appear to be much, if any, difference between the time providers spend with new versus established patients (Figure 25).

Once again, we apply a significance test and find that, in fact, this is true (Figure 26).

Another very important tool in the analyze phase is the cause-and-effect tool found in the Ishikawa (or fishbone) diagram. What our analysis has shown is that the most influential driver behind total cycle time (and wait time) occurs among new patients in the waiting room.

In Chapter 5, we discussed the steps for developing and using a fishbone diagram in detail. Figure 27 is an example of one that was created for this example.

Note the variability in some of the suggested causes compared with the similarity in others. For example, time of visit, scheduling, and "patient late" might be able to be combined into similar categories while issues with insurance validation or the use of unnecessary or duplicate forms would not. After every suggestion that could be made was made, the practice went back and reviewed each one and eliminated those that were determined to be noncontributory. Some of these may have included scheduling, insurance validation,

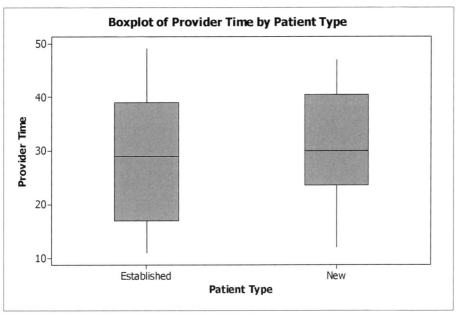

FIGURE 25. Boxplot of provider time.

Two-Sample T-Test and CI

```
Sample    N   Mean   StDev   SE Mean
1         75  27.2   10.7      1.2
2         75  28.9   11.5      1.3


Difference = mu (1) - mu (2)
Estimate for difference:  -1.64
95% CI for difference:  (-5.23, 1.95)
T-Test of difference = 0 (vs not =): T-Value = -0.90
P-Value = 0.368  DF = 147
```

FIGURE 26. Significance test of the difference between the mean values.

time of visit, and patient timeliness. It boiled down to the amount of time it took new patients to complete the intake forms. In order to assess this further, the practice conducted a series of small tests designed around the time issue. This is a good time to make an important point: quite often, the results of the cause-and-effect task will result in the need to conduct additional studies to validate and test the significance of your assumptions and to establish a baseline for comparison.

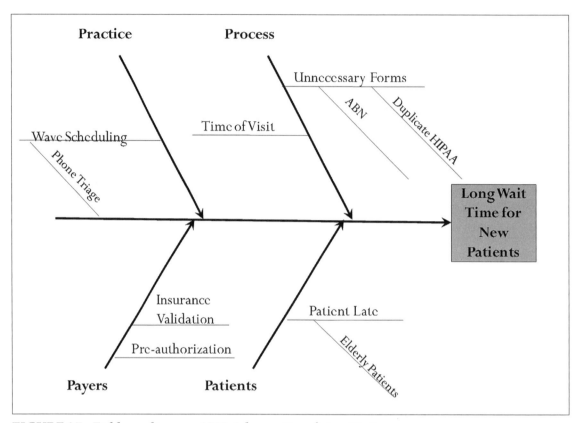

FIGURE 27. Fishbone diagram. ABN, Advance Beneficiary Notice.

In this case, the practice selected a small group of new patients at random, and for a week the practice timed the number of minutes it took new patients to complete the intake package, the number of times a new patient would ask a question about one or more of the documents, what questions were asked, and how many times each question was asked.

Another case involves a practice conducting a denial analysis. To begin, it tracked the total number of claim lines that were presented to the practice as denials, meaning that the payer denied payment due to any one of a number of reasons. To calculate the denial rate, the practice divided the total number of claim lines denied divided by the total claim lines submitted. The study was retroactive for 12 months and listed the metrics by week for the entire year. A run chart of the results is shown in Figure 28.

The purpose of visualizing the results was to determine whether there were any patterns, such as unusual trending, clusters of data points, etc. The above run chart shows a pretty normal distribution of data points. This indicated that the variability associated with denial percentages was likely due to normal variation and not any specific cause, in general.

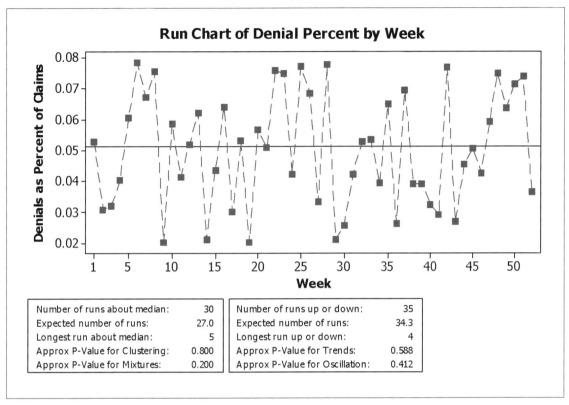

FIGURE 28. Denial rates per week.

The next step was to create a Pareto chart to determine the distribution of reason codes associated with the denials (Figure 29).

Of the 5.6% of denied claim lines, approximately 25% were the result of reason codes associated with an invalid code; 14% were due to documentation issues; 11% for non-covered services; and 9% due to NCCI violations. The Pareto chart continues to assign a distribution for the reason codes associated with denials, and when we reach the point at which about 80% of the reason codes are covered, we have, in a sense, created our marching orders. In our example here, the top 80% would include those denied due to wrong demographics.

From a structured perspective, we would likely begin with the most contributory of the buckets, which are invalid codes. To complete the analyze phase, the practice created a fishbone diagram with invalid codes as the main factor, and then went through a brainstorming session to identify the likely causes. As you can imagine, reasons like outdated code books, inability to update codes in the PMS, human error, and others were suggested.

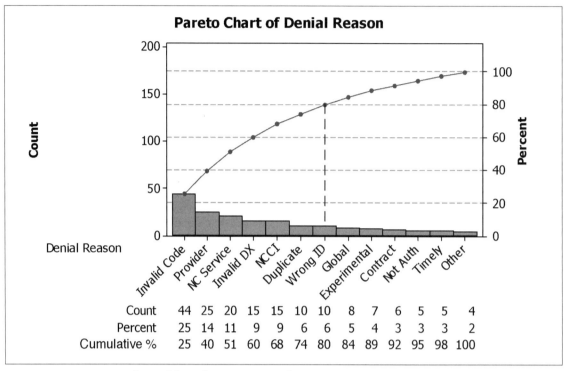

FIGURE 29.   Pareto chart of denial reason. Doc, documentation; DX, diagnosis; NC, noncovered; NCCI, National Correct Coding Initiative.

Improve

> *Man cannot use the same thinking to solve problems that he used to create them.*
>
> —ALBERT EINSTEIN

Having conducted a thorough analysis of the process in question and having identified the cause and effect as well as areas of potential waste, we are ready to begin to look at possible solutions. The purpose of the improve phase is to pick the best solutions from the list of possibilities, testing each for reasonableness, potential, and risk.

The steps normally followed in the improve step are:

- Generate potential solutions.
- Select the best of the bunch.
- Assess the benefits and the risks.
- Test your solutions.
- Implement those that meet the gold standard.

And the tools that are normally employed are:

- Negative brainstorming;
- Assumption busting;
- Error proofing;
- Brainstorming;
- Prioritization matrix;
- Solution screening;
- Pilot studies; and
- Hypothesis testing.

Please see the Chapter 5 for more information on these tools.

Discoveries: The Patient Visit Cycle

Let's spend some time looking again at our patient visit cycle time case study to get a better understanding of the improve phase of our DMAIC project. During the analysis, we determined that the primary driver behind excessive patient visit cycle time was waiting room time for new patients. The associated collateral problems this created included inefficient use of and scheduling for exam rooms, which backed up all patients; increases in cancellations (due to frustration over visit time); and walkouts (from waiting too long in the waiting room). These are all drivers of revenue, which was being negatively affected.

During the root cause analysis, the staff determined that the new patient intake package was not organized well and it contained unnecessary forms, such as Advance Beneficiary Notice (ABN) (whether or not the patient was covered by Medicare) and a duplicate HIPAA form (all patients signed a HIPAA form at check-in as well as receiving it in the new patient package). This resulted in patients taking too long to complete the paperwork; and even if they showed up early, as requested (11% did not), they still did not enter the active visit portion of the cycle on time.

The practice returned to the testing phase, and for a week, timed how long it took for new patients to complete the existing package in order to establish a baseline for comparison against the new benchmark goal. Now the practice was ready to begin the improve stage in earnest.

Solution Screening

During another brainstorming session (this tool is used a lot), the practice concluded that there were two strategies that would most likely resolve the problem: reengineering the intake package and finding a way to get patients to complete the package in advance. To accomplish this most efficiently, one group was assigned the redesign work and another to study the different ways in which advance work could be done most effectively.

The redesign team, using data from the test on the types and frequency of questions reported by patients, decided to test a typeface that was larger and more block-like, eliminating any italicized words. They also eliminated certain forms, such as the HIPAA and ABN forms. The latter was valid only for Medicare patients; used only 3% of the time (even less on new patients); and, due to Medicare rules, could not be kept on file. In all, three different package designs were proposed, and these were tested with a small group of patients, similar to what is discussed in the PDSA sections of this chapter that follow.

It is interesting to note that in most improvement projects, our hypothesized improvements will often reveal surprises regarding unsuspected results. For example, in order to reduce the number of pages in the intake form, the staff decided to print front-to-back. One of the unexpected consequences was this: when the patients, using a top-locked clipboard, turned the page (up), they lost the support of the clipboard for that page. To resolve this, the practice needed either to go back to a one-up printing method or get rid of the clipboards. The practice chose the latter, replacing them with three-ring binders, which, again unexpectedly, were much better received by the patients.

The second team, directed to find a way to get patients to complete the package in advance, came to four possible solutions:
1. E-mail the package as a .pdf file
2. Post the package as either a download or as forms on the practice's Web site
3. Mail the package to patients in advance of their appointment
4. Have a staff member call patients and complete the package on the phone via an interview process

While included with the redesign as part of a total solution, the decision process was a bit more complex and involved more subjectivity on behalf of the staff, so they decided to employ a decision matrix to assist with the decision (Figure 30).

In this case, because there were more issues involving compliance, staff involvement, and potential cost, the practice chose seven criteria for weighting. As expected, the redesign option was top on the list and was included more as a formality since work had already been done to improve that task. Regarding the other four possibilities, the matrix clearly revealed that having staff members interview the new patients was at the bottom of the list while the other three all occupied a relatively close position. Resolution would re-

Criteria (1 - 10, Agree - Disagree)	Redesign Intake Package	E-mail as .pdf	Internet Access	Snail Mail	Interview on Phone	Weight (1 - 10)
Implemented quickly	8	10	8	9	3	7
Solve the problem completely	8	5	5	5	7	10
Will not negatively impact patient	10	7	10	7	8	6
Will not negatively impact staff	7	10	10	6	3	6
No regulatory risks	8	10	10	10	10	8
Will not compromise quality	10	6	6	8	8	5
Will not cost more than $1,000	10	10	3	7	2	3
Weighted Value	382	362	345	332	283	

FIGURE 30. Decision matrix on intake package redesign.

quire a pilot study, whereby additional testing would be conducted to assess some of the primary risk areas, and then the staff would reassess the options based on the results of these tests.

Pilot Testing

Pilot testing involves looking at potential solutions with an analytic eye. The goal is to pick the best solution from a group of viable alternatives and to do so by creating a sort of simulation in advance. This can be done using both qualitative and quantitative methods. For example, to determine the best intake package, the staff rolled out three different versions and conducted a test of total time to completion and frequent questions in relation to each. The winner scored the best in that it took the shortest time to complete and required the fewest questions by patients.

Pilot studies help to validate the effectiveness of the solution as well as uncover potential risks that may not have been initially considered. They help with getting buy-in from upper management as well as process owners, particularly when the tests are very positive. From a management perspective, pilot studies can help to create probability models that result in lower overall risk; particularly of implementing an expensive solution that, ultimately, doesn't work. The latter is similar to a builder's motto of "Measure twice, cut once." One of the great advantages of pilot testing is that it can be controlled to allow for isolation of factors, which allows you to observe individual effects, such as for type size, wording, or paragraph placement. Pilot tests can also be quantified through hypothesis testing, which allows the team to make projections (or to infer the results) to a larger base, such as practice- or enterprise-wide organizational activity.

As discussed, redesigning the intake package became a no-brainer, and testing the changes was relatively simple. Remember, this was a highly focused task with minimal risk. Moving up a level, the practice started to investigate the different possible solutions to have the package filled out in advance and then brought in completed by the patient. Again, these were an advance e-mail with the intake package attached as a .pdf file, the ability to either download or complete forms from the practice's Web site, or mailing the package to patients via U.S. Postal Service.

Of the above three, two share one common delivery method: access to the Internet, either solely using an e-mail product or a Web browser. This created a need to quantify the volume of potential new patients that had access to this technology. The practice created a short questionnaire that asked the following questions:

- Do you have access to the Internet?
- How comfortable are you with your ability to browse the Internet?
- Do you have access to e-mail?
- How often do you check your e-mail?
- Do you have a printer?

From the surveys they sent out, they selected a group of patients that had Internet access and regularly checked their e-mail, and asked them the following questions:

- How comfortable would you be entering your health information on a Web site?
- How likely would you be to print out forms from an e-mail?

The results surprised the administrator, who was a younger, technically competent person. To put this in context, the practice was located in a rural area and had a fairly large elderly population.

Of those surveyed, 51% stated they had access to the Internet, including e-mail. It's interesting to note that a small percentage of respondents actually did not know what the Internet was and stated so. Of the 51% that stated they had access to the Internet, 58% said they would be somewhat or very comfortable completing the forms on a Web site. This means that the maximum likelihood for participation would be around 25%, well below the threshold set by the practice.

Of the 51% that had Internet access, 62% said they checked their e-mail at least once a week, which means that the maximum likelihood for participation would be around 30%. Even more informative was that of this 62%, 21% either didn't know if they had a printer or reported not having a printer, which reduced the probability even more.

As a result, the practice decided to scrap the idea of using electronic communication to resolve this issue as the investment in time and resources would likely not return

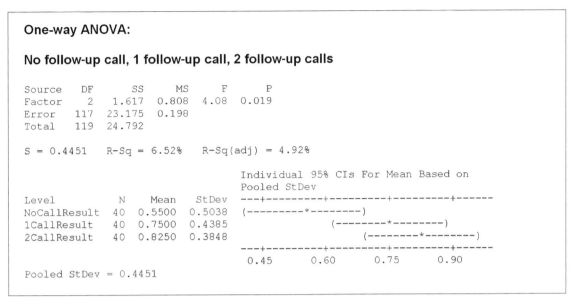

```
One-way ANOVA:

No follow-up call, 1 follow-up call, 2 follow-up calls

Source     DF      SS      MS     F      P
Factor      2    1.617   0.808  4.08  0.019
Error     117   23.175   0.198
Total     119   24.792

S = 0.4451   R-Sq = 6.52%   R-Sq(adj) = 4.92%

                                   Individual 95% CIs For Mean Based on
                                   Pooled StDev
Level           N     Mean    StDev  ---+---------+---------+---------+------
NoCallResult   40   0.5500   0.5038  (---------*--------)
1CallResult    40   0.7500   0.4385               (---------*--------)
2CallResult    40   0.8250   0.3848                      (--------*--------)
                                       ---+---------+---------+---------+------
                                         0.45      0.60      0.75      0.90

Pooled StDev = 0.4451
```

FIGURE 31. **One-way ANOVA: No-call results, one-call results, and two-call results.**

enough of a benefit to warrant the fix. Instead, it decided to focus on snail mail as a possible solution. What was clear to all was that every patient had a physical address and had access to postal mail.

The practice developed a test to see if mailing the package in advance would work, and it took into consideration suggestions that one or two follow-up calls would be required to improve the rate of response. As such, the practice decided to mail a package to all new patients scheduled over the next month, and with the following differences:

- One-third would receive a reminder call (to complete the package) three days in advance of the appointment.
- One-third would receive two calls: one three days prior and one the day prior to the appointment.
- One-third of scheduled new patients would receive no reminder call.

The practice conducted an ANOVA test, and Figure 31 shows the results of the test.

The study revealed that while there wasn't a statistically significant difference between no reminder call and one reminder call, there was between no reminder call and two reminder calls. Notice, however, that the CIs are quite large, and, in this case, were due to an inadequate sample. Also note that the results for one call were virtually the same as for two calls. Since this was not designed to be a statistically valid random sample, but rather a test to create an action point, the practice opted to mail a package and make one reminder call three days prior to the appointment date.

Control

> *A man is like a fraction whose numerator is what he is and*
> *whose denominator is what he thinks of himself. The larger*
> *the denominator, the smaller the fraction.*
>
> —Leo Tolstoy

The final phase in the DMAIC platform is the Control phase. The control phase exists to monitor how successfully the implemented improvements have been integrated into the practice itself. The goals of the control phase are to assess the final process capability, revisit the process with an eye for sustaining the project, evaluate methods for defect prevention, explore various methods to monitor the process, and implement a control plan, which includes integration into the practice framework.

The steps in the control phase are:

- Quantify the improvement.
- Implement ongoing measurement.
- Standardize the solutions.
- Integrate into the organization.
- Close the project.

Let's take a close look at each of these steps before listing the most often used tools.

Quantify the Improvement

The main purpose of this step is to show whether the goal has been met. In our prior example, the practice reassessed the metrics after 90 days, and found that 81% of all new patients were completing the package in advance, which resulted in a reduction in overall wait time for new patients from 51 to 33 minutes. While a significant improvement, it was still six minutes less than the original goal of 27 minutes. Factoring all patients in the practice, it reduced the overall cycle time for a visit episode by approximately 22 minutes. Walk-outs were nearly nonexistent, and no-shows and cancellations were reduced by 61% and 77%, respectively.

Overall, among the three physicians, the practice was able to schedule (and see) an additional nine patients per day. With an average revenue-to-visit ratio of $122, this translated into $285,480 in additional revenue each year, which, subtracting the variable expense, translated into over $250,000 to the bottom line.

Implement Ongoing Measurement

Being able to track the improvement beyond the initial assessment is critical for long-term benefits. This involves establishing a policy on how ongoing measurements will be conducted. Which steps will be measured and at what intervals will this occur? Who is responsible, and to whom will the results be presented? What thresholds will be in place so that if the process variability gets too large, it will be subject to review? In our case study here, the practice determined to sample wait time and package completion percent on 10% of new patients per month, while metrics on walkouts and revisit cancellations would be conducted on 10% of established patients each month.

Standardize the Solutions

This involves educating staff, management, and often patients as to the new process or the improvements that have been implemented. The benefit of standardizing the solution focuses on the "everyone on the same page" concept. It is always frustrating for any business when, after an improvement has been implemented, some people continue to do things the old way while others participate in the new-and-improved way. Standardization requires that the new process maps are available and understood by all affected parties. It means that someone in the organization needs to create a written policy and/or procedure that becomes part of the policy and procedure manual for the practice. It means that all new employees are trained on, understand, and sign-off on the current state of the process with an understanding toward continued improvement.

Standardizing a process allows employees to maintain greater control over processes for which they are involved. It also allows all employees and management to measure effectiveness against benchmarks and so-called "standards." Good projects, those that result in process improvements, should have polymorphic characteristics. This means that the steps used in this project should work for other process improvement projects as well. Remember, what you are doing is building a model for solutions rather than just the solutions themselves. And in a good model, any number of potential solutions can be incorporated. Standardization allows for comparative analyses that can be used to measure long-term changes and pinpoint special cause variations that might not be picked up on a shorter-term run. This task also helps to ensure that, even after the project team disbands and members leave the organization, new staff can pick up where the former staff left off. Remember, the goal is long-term survival of a working process improvement plan.

Organization Integration

By all measures, if the project was a success (remember, this was defined at the very beginning), it should be written into policy. The new process should be seen as the new standard operating procedure (SOP) rather than treated as just another change or fix. The key here is that it is written documentation rather than anecdote or folklore passed down from one generation to another. The practice might also want to consider formal communications about the policy, such as visual presentations, educational workshops, etc. The more critical personnel involved, such as process owners and team members, the better.

Quite often, we see a new administrator or department manager hired in a practice who brings along his or her own way of doing things. If improvements are not integrated into the framework of the business, it is very easy for newcomers to "not see" the improvements and begin to implement their own ideas of how things should work without the benefit of understanding what already works. If it ain't broke, don't fix it! Since politics plays a role in nearly every organization, it is important to have key political and influential players on board. This will also help with getting approval for future projects.

Close the Project

Once again, this might seem like a given but you might be amazed at how often this doesn't happen, at least not formally. Every project, whether successful or not, should have a well-defined point of closure. This should have been worked out in the Define phase under the project charter. It helps to develop a "storyboard" of sorts that includes a checklist of each DMAIC phase of the project. Doing so presents a clear and present target that, when reached, automatically signals that the project has ended. This should include summaries, conclusions, control plans, etc.

Make certain that all records and documentation are clear and available for review by all players. And while the documentation might be indifferent to the tactical components, it should clearly outline the strategic goals and how (and if) they were met. If the project was not considered a success, the documentation should detail why it failed and what the team plans to do to either abandon or reestablish the goals. This documentation is absolutely critical for long-term survival. Finally, develop a closure action log, which includes a policy for handing over the project to the stakeholders.

Control Phase Tools

There are two primary categories of tools in the control phase: the first dealing with statistical process control (SPC) charts and graphs, and the second, control plans. The SPC category includes control charts, time series charts, run charts, trend analyses, and the like. The control plans are broken down into five phases: training, documentation, monitoring, response, and aligning the systems and structures. These will be discussed in greater detail shortly.

Once again, I face the challenge here of explaining the importance of a topic that, like the areas on data and statistics, exceeds the scope of this book. I will, however, discuss the basic characteristics of SPC, using examples from actual improvement projects to illustrate the benefits of including these in the control phase.

SPC charts, or just control charts, are time-series like graphs that contain upper and lower control limits. Unlike specification limits, which define the goal of a process, control charts measure the variability within a process to determine whether it is in or out of "control." This can get a bit confusing for more complex systems, but the crux is this: you are using the method to determine whether your process is subject to something other than normal variability.

In our wait time example, we expect that there will be variability around an average wait time but when a "blip" occurs that is outside of the control criteria (say, two standard deviations from the mean or a trend up or down), it sends a clear signal that something unique has happened that affects the process as a whole. Therefore, how well the process stays within those control limits determines whether, if, and how well a process is in control.

There are two key components of SPC charts: historical and concurrent. Historical charts review a given period of time (retroactively) that are then used to determine overall stability. Often, these are used to benchmark a process. Concurrent analysis is a more real-time analysis of process performance that enables the practice to detect and react to process problems immediately or nearly immediately. We often see these methods combined, for example, looking at the history of a process over the past six months (prior to any change or implementation of an improvement) and then comparing with the seventh month to see whether the implementation of a fix or improvement has, in fact, affected the control characteristics of the process.

The I-MR Chart. One of the more common types of control charts found in medical practices is called the I-MR, or Individuals-Moving Range, chart. Individual values (I) and moving range (MR) charts are used when each measurement represents one or one metric group. The subgroup size is equal to one when I-MR charts are used since there is no definition for sub-groups, such as we might find when looking at conversion factor values for a provider segmented into major and minor coding (or code) categories. These charts are very simple to prepare and use. The graphic shows the individuals chart in which

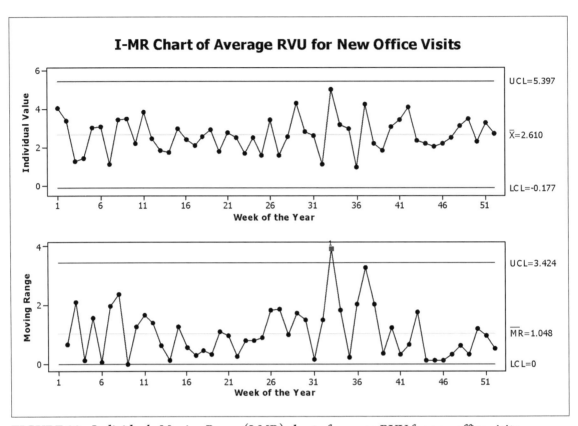

FIGURE 32. Individuals-Moving Range (I-MR) chart of average RVU for new office visits.

the individual measurement values are plotted with the centerline being the average of the individual measurements. The moving range chart shows the range between two subsequent measurements.

There are certain situations when opportunities to collect data are limited or when grouping the data into subgroups simply doesn't make sense. Perhaps the most obvious of these cases is when each individual measurement is already a rational subgroup. This might happen when the measurements are widely spaced in time or when only one measurement is available in evaluating the process. Such situations include monthly revenue figures, provider productivity ratios, E/M coding differentials, etc. All of these situations indicate a subgroup size of one. Because this type of chart is dealing with individual measurements, it is not as sensitive as other types of control charts in detecting process changes.

Note that in Figure 32, which looks at the average RVU for new office visits (possibly for one provider or specialty), while the individual measurements appear in control, there is a point at week 33 where the average between the prior weeks reported an out-of-control

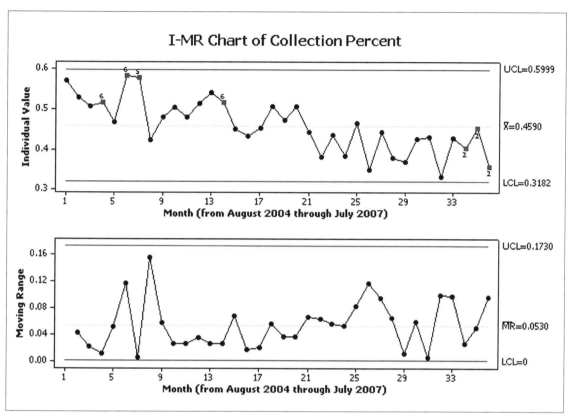

FIGURE 33. IM-R chart of collection percent.

point. In this case, the test for any point greater than three standard deviations from the mean failed.

The I-MR chart shown in Figure 33 reviews monthly collections for a provider over a period of three years.

In this example, three tests failed, including having nine points in a row on the same side of the center line (may indicate a trend); two out of three points more than two standard deviations from the mean; and four out of five points more than one standard deviation from the mean. Each of these tests would indicate that there was something besides normal variability causing this to occur. In the above Individual value chart, it is easy to see that there is a downward trend with historical markers in the beginning and concurrent markers in the last three months.

Relating back to our example of wait time, the chart in Figure 34 identifies specific moments when something occurred during a given day over a three-month period that caused the process to report an out-of-control moment.

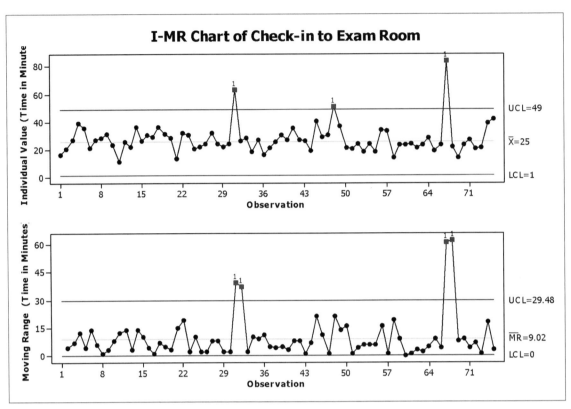

FIGURE 34. I-MR chart of check-in to exam room time.

Note that in the individual value chart, there are three points that have failed a control test with all three representing a data point that was more than three times the standard deviation. From a control phase perspective, the practice went back to each of those individual days to see what caused this to occur. If, for example, it was an isolated incident, such as a medical emergency calling the physician away or, in the case of day 66, a loss of power for several hours, the practice can simply develop a contingency plan for when these types of things happen. If, however, those moments were to indicate a pattern of change, it would signal the practice to begin another look at the process. Since a business is constantly in a state of flux and dynamics are normally fluid, it is not uncommon to find ourselves revisiting a process that now requires additional work to keep up to date with those dynamics.

The U Chart. Another type of chart that is commonly found in a medical practice is called a U chart, which is used to plot specific errors within a process or a task. A classic example has to do with E/M coding. Many of the E/M codes require either two or three key com-

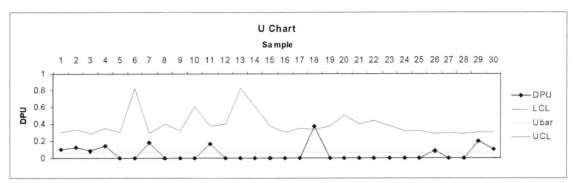

FIGURE 35. U chart of number of errors per claim for each day's processing of claim forms. Ubar represents the average of the subgroup defects (or errors) per unit (weighted average if the subgroup sizes are different). DPU represents the number of defects (in this case, errors) per unit (in this case, per claim).

ponents (past family/social history, physician exam, and medical decision making) to be present for that category (i.e., office visits or hospital visits). Each of these key components has its own ranking system, and the sum of the positions of the ranks for each category is used to determine the appropriate code level. Therefore, in a chart audit, it is as, if not more important to understand whether errors were made within each of the individual key methods as opposed to just determining if there is a match on the procedure code as a whole. The "U" in U chart stands for "units" and refers to the errors per unit of service; in our case, the number of errors discovered for each of the key components when coding an E/M chart.

Another example has to do with looking at the possible range of errors that can occur on something more complex, such as a claim form. Defects on insurance claim forms are a problem for many medical practices. Every claim line form has to be checked and corrected before being transmitted to the payer. When completing an 837 (electronic claim), a particular practice may have to populate hundreds of fields, including patient demographics, ICD-9 and procedure codes, authorization numbers, etc. A blank or incorrect field is an error, and any one could result in a denial or up-front rejection of the claim, requiring rework and adding to the cost of the process.

The graph in Figure 35 shows a practice that tracked its claims performance by calculating the number of errors per claim for each day's processing of claim forms. The graph demonstrates their performance on a U chart.

The general procedure for U charts is as follows:
1. Determine purpose of the chart.
2. Select data collection point.
3. Establish basis for subgrouping.

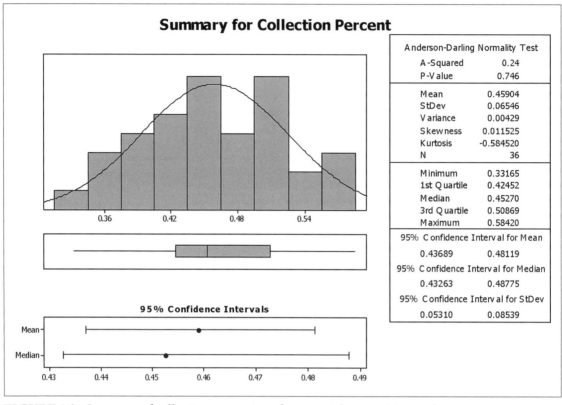

FIGURE 36. Summary of collection percentage for a provider over 36 months.

4. Establish sampling interval and determine sample size.
5. Set up forms for recording and charting data and write specific instructions on use of the chart.
6. Collect and record data.
7. Count the number of nonconformities for each of the subgroups.
8. Input into Excel or other statistical software.
9. Interpret chart together with other pertinent sources of information on the process, and take corrective action if necessary.

Time Series Analyses. A time series analysis is an analysis of the movement of a process over a period of time. A time series plot, well, plots that data into a visual graphic display. Time series charts are very important for understanding the change in behavior of any set of data over any given period of time. The following is a good example as to why you would want to use a time series chart. The purpose of this project was to assess the feasibility of purchasing A/R from the physician as part of a buyout. The physician reported average

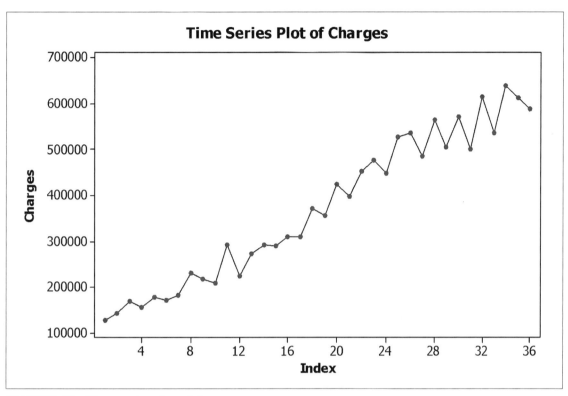

FIGURE 37. **Time series plot of charges.**

charge days in A/R of 60, meaning that the average time between date of service and final payment was approximately 60 days. As a result, the physician wanted to sell his most recent 60 days' worth of charges to the practice based on his assessment of his gross revenues as a percent of collection during the most recent 36-month period.

In Figure 36, note that the average collections as a percent of charges is around 46%, and as such, the physician wanted to sell the practice his last two months of charges (just under $400,000) for $184,000, or 45% of that amount.

He even produced his own set of time series graphs for charges and collections, as shown in Figures 37 and 38.

The initial impression is that charges and revenue seem to be trending upwards at about the same rate, indicating that the ratio between the two is likely constant. But look at the range of values on the Y axis of the chart. Charges go from $100,000 to $700,000 while revenue goes from $100,000 to $300,000. This is a great way to lie with statistics; comparing graphs with different magnitudes on either axis. When plotted together, the graph looked like Figure 39.

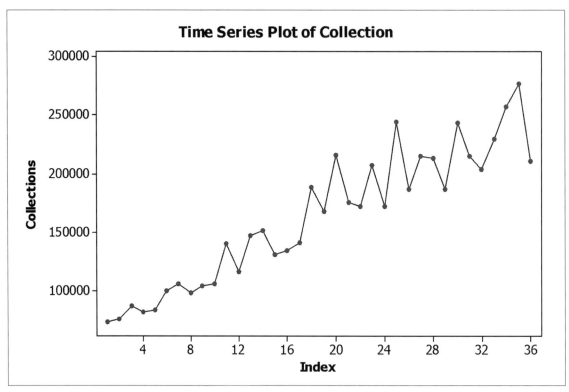

FIGURE 38.   Time series plot of collections.

Note that, when presented properly, it shows that revenues are growing at a much slower pace, perhaps even stalling near the end of this cycle. Plotting revenues as a percent of charges (Figure 40) painted the most striking picture of what was actually happening.

Note that this gives a much clearer picture of the value of the A/R, with the last month's collection at around 36% rather than the average of 46%.

Another way to view a time series chart is the use of a rolling average. This is particularly good for smoothing out data sets with large amounts of variability or those that are tending toward a dynamic trend. In our example, it would be important in order to assess the plateaus of collection percentages over grouped periods in order to try to assess the value of the charge A/R over a more recent yet balanced time period.

Figure 41 shows what a rolling average plot would look like if the periods were aggregated into six-month groups.

Note that this shows a normalization of the downward trend during the past six or seven months. It also allows the practice to assess more accurately the value of the A/R, which, in this case, amounts to around 40%.

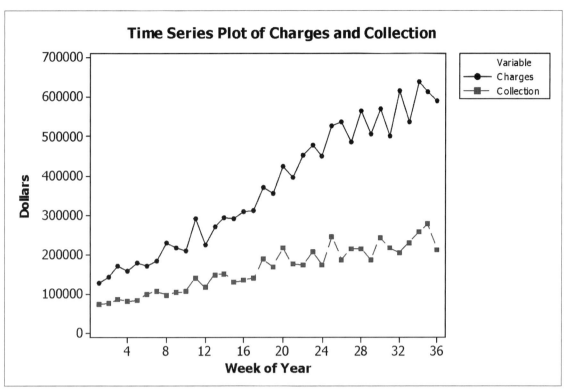

FIGURE 39. Time series plot of charges and collections.

One other unique type of time series analysis is called a time and trend graph. This not only shows the changes over time but can also predict (with a varying degree of accuracy) what may happen in the future. The trend graph makes use of regression analysis, or least means squared (LMS), techniques to calculate the slope of a line and then extend it out into the future. Remember, though—and this is critically important—very few procedures continue on in a linear fashion forever. Take a look at the chart in Figure 42.

Here, we have predicted out another 12 months to try to estimate what the percent collection ratio might be if it were to continue in a linear fashion. The problem, however, arises when the projections conflict with reality. If we were to believe this trend, we might find that, at some point, the physician would be billing $1,000,000 a month and collecting nothing.

Run Charts. The final chart to discuss here is the run chart, which is, in effect, nothing more than a time series chart with a different set of statistical tests that allow you to understand the significance of things like trends, oscillation, clusters, and mixtures. A run

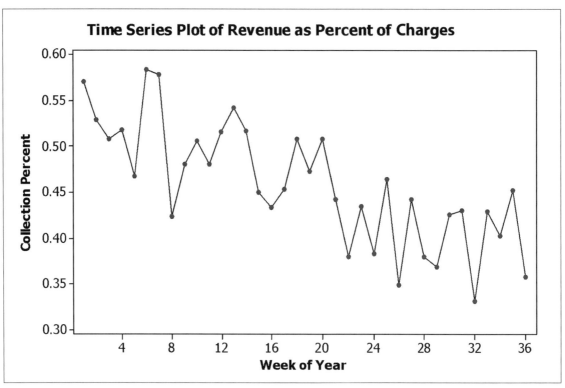

FIGURE 40.   Time series plot of revenues as a percent of charges.

chart won't look much different from a standard time series chart with the exception of the additional information that is provided, as seen in Figure 43.

This plots the average conversion factor for new office visits for a provider over a 52-week period. At week 26, the practice brought in a trainer to assist the physician with coding, and the graphic shows the 26 weeks prior to and the 26 weeks after the training. Overall, the analysis showed no clustering, no trends, and no statistically significant patterns of oscillation. The visual allows us to see that, after the training, variability seemed to be more equally distributed around the mean, although this is not a measurement of randomness.

The Control Plan.   Finally, at the close of a project, the control plan should be put into place. As stated before, it is very important to have rigorous data collection in place before a project can be closed. If this does not occur, it is likely the process will revert within a short period of time. As with our data collection plan, it includes documenting the "who," "what," "how," "where," and "when" of data collection on the back end of the project. This is best achieved through the use of some type of formal control plan, many examples of which can be found by searching the Internet. The control plan template defines the char-

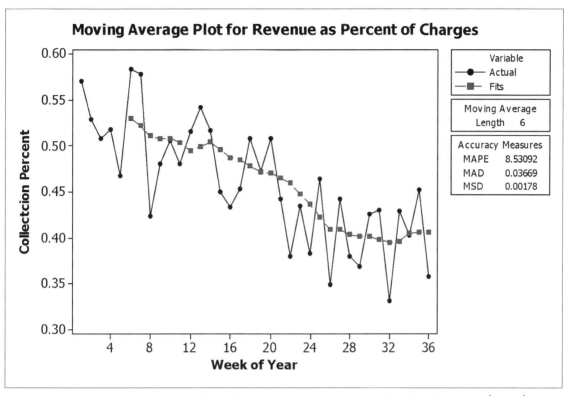

FIGURE 41. Moving average plot for collection percent. The mean absolute deviation (MAD) measures the accuracy of fitted time series values. It expresses accuracy in the same units as the data, which helps conceptualize the amount of error. Mean absolute percentage error (MAPE) measures the accuracy of fitted time series values. It expresses accuracy as a percentage. The mean squared deviation (MSD) is always computed using the same denominator, n, regardless of the model, so you can compare MSD values across models. MSD is a more sensitive measure than MAD of an unusually large forecast error.

acteristics that are measured, specifications, historical capability, methodology, and how to respond if and when the process is out of control.

Figure 44 is a basic example of what a stock control plan template might look like:

Section 1 shows the basic demographics of the project while section 2 contains the hierarchy for authority and approval of the project itself. Section 3 is an organizational component that allows proper tracking and revision control of the plan. Section 4 describes the processes and any subprocesses (similar to steps or tasks) while section 5 reports the key input and output variables or metrics. Section 6 is used to define any specification characteristics, such as might be found when considering compliance risk, and section 7 is used to define the target as well as the lower and upper specification limits. In the case of our waiting time case study, we might put 27 minutes in as the target with a lower spec of 0

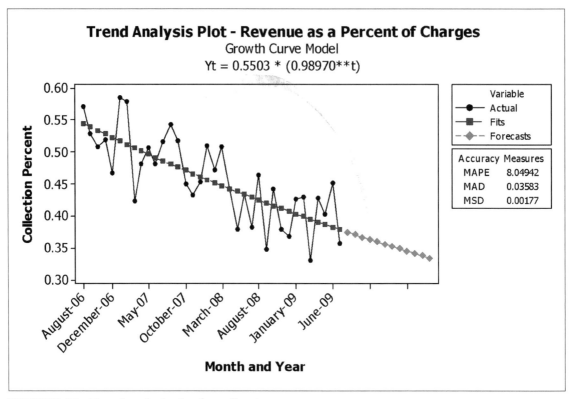

FIGURE 42. Trend analysis plot for collection percent.

(we don't want to limit how quickly we see a patient) and an upper spec limit of 35, meaning that anytime wait time exceeds 35 minutes, we will take a look to see what caused this to happen. Section 8 lists the different metrics, including methods and roles. Finally, section 9 might define the threshold for taking action and what action was taken as well as where in the policy and procedure document the change will be recorded.

Again, remember that this is a simple generic example, and it is always important to customize the template for your organization as well as for your group.

PDSA/PDCA

Often referred to as the Deming cycle (or Deming wheel), PDSA/PDCA stands for Plan, Do, Study (or Check), and Act. Its origins as PDCA is normally credited to statistician Walter A. Shewhart, back in the 1920s. Renowned statistician and quality improvement guru W. Edwards Deming modified the Shewhart cycle, replacing the "C" for "check" with "S" for "study." They are both pretty much the same thing, and we often see them used interchangeably.

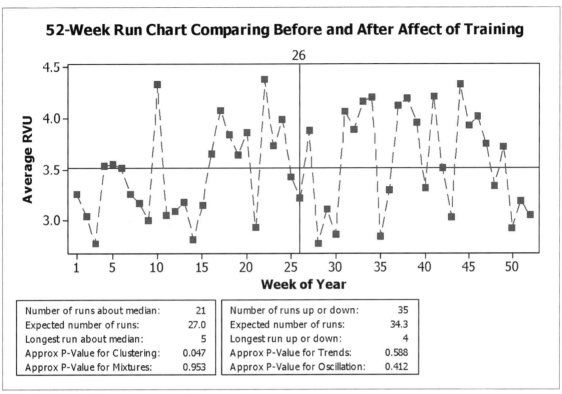

FIGURE 43. Average conversion factor for new office visits for a provider over a 52-week period.

Deming-type models such as these are designed around the idea of continuous improvement, and this is a bit more important than some people seem to realize. I am sure that, in your organization, you can point to some process improvement project that was initiated and even carried out that may not have been considered a formal "process improvement" project. Many times, we look at these projects as one-time efforts directed toward a specific issue or problem, and when it is solved (or we think it is solved), we go back to business as usual.

Newton's first law of motion states that an object at rest tends to stay at rest, and an object in motion tends to stay in motion with the same speed and in the same direction unless acted upon by an unbalanced force. In essence, it takes more energy to get an object from rest into motion, and often more energy to get an object in motion to stop. From the perspective of continuous process improvement, it requires less energy to maintain a commitment to continuous improvement than to start and stop, depending on identification of a particular issue. In essence, we want to create an environment for process improvement that is continuous in that it is a philosophy of vigilance. We are always looking forward

Process Name:					Prepared by:						Page: of		
Customer: **(1)**					Approved by: **(2)**						Document #: **(3)**		
Location:					Approved by:						Revision Date:		
Area:					Approved by:						Supercedes:		
Subprocess	Subprocess Step	CTS		Specification Characteristic	Specification Requirement			Measurement Method	Sample Size	Frequency	Who Measures	Where Recorded	Decision Rule/ Corrective Action	SOP Reference
		KPIV	KPOV		LSL	Target	USL							
(4)		**(5)**		**(6)**	**(7)**				**(8)**				**(9)**	

FIGURE 44. Stock control plan template. CTS, critical to success; KPIV, key process input variables; KPOV, key process output variables; LSL, lower specification limit; SOP, standard operating procedure; USL, upper specification limit.

to the next project because, in reality, there are always constraints and always issues that work against efficiency; and for all of us, there remain always opportunities for improvements. That is one of the reasons that I don't like so-called standards that define what constitutes "best practice" measurements. For example, best practice might be A/R between 25 and 35 days. For many, this means that when they hit that range, they stop working to improve when it might be possible to reduce A/R as far as 15 days.

Why Use PDSA?

Many of us are resistant to more formalized tasking when it comes to process improvement. So often, solving a problem "feels" intuitive, and we rely on experience and intuition to find a solution. When it works (and it often does), without the benefit of documenting what we did and how we did it, we rob ourselves of the opportunity to create a model for improvement that, in the future, would prove to be more effective and efficient.

PDSA is nowhere near as formal as some of the other platforms, DMAIC in particular. PDSA presents us with a low-risk way of trying out ideas. The concept is, "It's a cinch by the inch," meaning that we take baby steps, evaluating benefits and risks at a very granular level. Because of its short cycle time, we are often able to determine relative effectiveness right away, knowing early on if there will be any benefit to our idea. Having a few rapid and inexpensive successes helps to build confidence in the team and makes buy-in from owners and upper management just that much easier. From a quality perspective, it helps to uncover problems early on, preventing them from reaching the customer. In beginning a PDSA project, there are three pertinent questions that need to be answered:

1. What are we trying to accomplish?
2. How will we know that a change has occurred and whether it is positive?
3. What changes can we make that will improve the situation or solve the problem?

Remember, PDSA is not a full-blown plan. PDSA projects are very small in scale, so if you are thinking in months, think in weeks; if you are thinking in weeks, think in days. If you are looking at the facility, look at a department; a department, look at a team. And if looking at a team, look at just one person to engage. The same is true of the target customers. If you are thinking all patients, think of a patient type, such as new or established. If thinking of a patient type, think of a small sample—maybe three to five patients to start.

Trial and Learning

Often, our projects are focused on trial and error, which ultimately results in chaos more often than not. Trial and error projects are usually directed by all action and no thinking. This is great if you have unlimited resources and can afford the cost of continual mistakes but most organizations are not in this boat. Making decisions on bad or no information usually results in bad decisions, which is something none of us can afford to have happen.

The other end of the spectrum is a detailed study. These are characterized by all thinking and no action. We plod through the data ad nauseam, and every time we get to an opportunity to act, we simply dive deeper into the study mode. There is simply too much planning and modeling and not enough action, and so often we end up with "paralysis of analysis"; we get hung up on the research and the data, and begin to lose our sense of direction and focus.

The ideal approach, using PDSA, is what is known as trial and learning. It takes the best of both worlds and leaves the rest on the outside. Trial and learning, as shown in Figure 45, is characterized by investigating, planning, and then developing an approach to solve the problem. Remember, when using PDSA, whatever it is you are looking at is NOT a research project. It's about small changes, and the data you gather are specific to that small change.

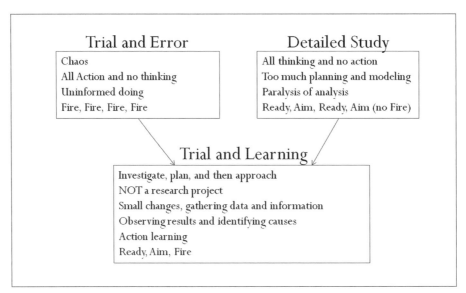

FIGURE 45. Trial and learning concept.

For example, if you are looking at dealing with waiting room time, instead of looking at average time for all patients, maybe you look at average time just for new patients. And even more granular, you look at waiting time just for new Medicare patients. And the data you collect looks only at how long it takes to complete the new patient package and how many (and what types) of questions those patients ask. Assuming homogeneity amongst this group, you look only at data for patients on one particular day. If you were doing a study, you would conduct a probe analysis, calculate the average wait time and standard deviation, and use that to identify a sample size. Then, you would stratify the sample by patient type, create a randomized technique and maybe (maybe!) a month later, you would have the data you needed to begin the project. This is NOT how PDSA works.

After collecting the minimal amount of data necessary, you observe the results and figure out the root cause (or causes). The key here is action learning; it's not only fixing or solving a problem or improving a process or increasing quality or reducing risk, it's about learning how to do it quickly and efficiently. In organizations that engage in a continuous model of using PDSA for these types of projects, problem solving becomes second nature, and they find themselves engaged without even thinking about it.

Implementing PDSA/PDCA

Figure 46 is a graphical representation of the flow for a PDSA/PDCA deployment model. Let's take a look at each of the steps in more detail.

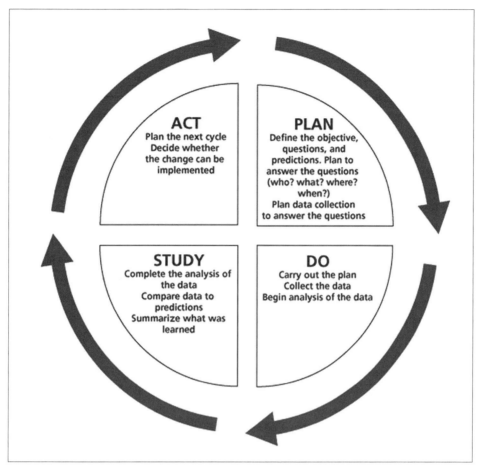

FIGURE 46. PDSA/PDCA deployment model.

Plan

The "Plan" phase (the "P" in "PDSA") gets you focused on the issue at hand. It is here that you define the purpose of the test. As such, there are seven questions you want to answer at the beginning of any PDSA project:

1. What is the purpose of the test?
2. What change idea are we trying to employ?
3. What will be the indicators of success?
4. How will data be collected?
5. What will be the sample size?
6. What is the time frame for each of the steps and to completion?
7. What do we hypothesize will happen?

Are you looking to find a better way to measure A/R? Are you trying to reduce MRI room turnaround time? Are you trying to cut five minutes off the patient visit cycle time? Maybe you want to find a more effective method to track denials; something that includes looking at reason codes by payer. You must also create the options of the change ideas you are considering trying. In essence, you are developing a hypothesis. You may, for example, hypothesize that certain payers have higher A/R because their edit rules are different, and your idea is to measure A/R for specific cases that involved multiple diagnoses codes and/or multiple modifiers. In one case, a practice was concerned about an increase in the number of denials that were related to NCCI edit policy and wanted to know whether there was any difference in this among payers. It believed that this might be isolated to a few payers and decided to see if it was true, and if so, if a meeting with those payers would help to resolve the problem.

What many practices (and businesses, for that matter) miss is defining what constitutes success. What needs to happen in order to determine if the project was successful? It may or may not be tied to the success of the intervention. For example, it may be that success is simply defined as discovering whether there is a problem, and then another PDSA project could ensue designed to deal with finding a solution on a larger scale, such as involvement of legal assistance or a state or national association.

Moving forward in the plan phase, you should determine how the data will be collected. In our example here, the practice decides to look at all denials with a reason code 97 and remark code M15, which often result when billing for an included NCCI edit pair. Data may be pulled directly from the PMS or, alternatively, it may require a manual review of EOBs. In any case, remember: small samples, short time frame.

Determining sample size can a bit more tricky and depends on the purpose and criticality of the analysis. While we want to avoid the paralysis of analysis problem that often occurs in detailed studies, we do not want to ignore the importance of scientific study as analytics remain at the core of successful projects. Just try to find a balance between sample size and time because if the PDSA can't jump start in a few days, it is likely to stall out and fail. Many of these types of projects can happen quickly, say within a week or so. I have rarely seen one go beyond 30 days without transforming into a different platform. Since we often learn more from being surprised, don't forget to make some assumptions about what you expect to happen as a result of your study.

Plan Action Steps.   As defined above, the first step is to identify the problem or question that will engage the project. The next step is to establish the team that will take on the project and involve the team from the beginning steps, including brainstorming sessions directed at designing the tactical, strategic, and logistical plans of action. Realistically, for smaller practices, the team may consist of just one or two people. Remember, while this is a great way to speed along decision making and reduce conflict, it also makes it nearly impossible to get fresh ideas on the table. If you don't have access to cross- or inter-disciplinary team members, consider a virtual team. Call others involved in process improvement or visit some of the list serves and ask people for input, advice, and help. It should also be noted that, in some organizations that are committed to process improvement activities, teams (or a single team) may have already been created and are in place waiting for improvement projects to originate.

One of the important functions of the team is to define the goal of the project; for example, to reduce A/R by seven days, or to shorten the patient visit cycle time by five minutes, or to perform three additional imaging procedures per day. The goal should be both realistic and achievable. Unrealistic goals, or those that require an inordinate amount of resources, or even those where the continued cost of the improvement is greater than the value of the improvement are often like teaching a pig how to fly. It won't happen, and it is frustrating and sometimes discouraging for the team.

The term we use to define the difference between where you are and where you want to be is "gap analysis," and it is a great tool for defining the level of granularity required to improve the process. For example, if you want to get A/R days to 40 and it is currently 45, it means that you don't have to worry about the 45 or the 40, just the 5 days that define the gap. We see the same with patient visit cycle time; if you want a reduction from 67 minutes to 60 minutes, you only need to figure out how to cut the 7 minutes from the cycle, not how to reengineer the practice to build a patient visit model that can see a patient through in 60 minutes. Often, once you begin to think in terms of gaps rather than absolutes, projects become less overwhelming, and more excitement can be generated by the team members.

The next step in this phase is to develop an intervention plan. This includes defining the steps and resources that will be required to close the gap and reach your goal. This may include resources like time, dollars, personnel, outside experts, new or upgraded technologies, etc. This can involve estimating the benefits because often a formal return-on-investment analysis will need to be prepared in order to get access to the approvals and resources necessary to move forward. Even though PDSA/PDCA platforms can be informal in their approach, it is still important to create and maintain a documentation trail along the way. This is useful when a project works (to see what was done correctly and how it can be applied to the next project) and when a project fails (to see what went wrong and avoid the same mistakes the next time around).

The tools you may use in this step include:

- Process Mapping;
- SIPOC;
- VOC;
- Brainstorming;
- Pareto Analysis;
- Priority Matrices; and
- Cause-and-Effect (Ishikawa or Fishbone) Diagrams.

Do

In the "Do" phase, you collect the data necessary to quantify the gaps and then go ahead and implement the change by carrying out your plan of action. Unless exhaustive alpha and beta testing has been done on the recommended solutions, it is important to be flexible, to be willing to make changes to your plan if, as you walk through it, you see that things are not working out as planned.

For example, in shortening the time it takes to get a patient in the door, seen, and back out the door, we decide to e-mail intake packages to new patients and discover that the percentage of patients completing the package in advance is so small that we need to re-think our strategy. In this case, maybe a reminder phone call a day or two prior to the visit will help to improve the number of patients that comply. Or perhaps we decided to refer delinquent claims to a collection agency earlier than before and discover that the collection ratios are no different than before yet the cost is greater, reducing profitability. In this case, we may decide to either bring the function back in house or renegotiate our agreement with the collection agency.

In the Plan step, your review may have been limited to process mapping, brainstorming the issues, and cause-and-effect activities. Here, you need to be able to measure (or quantify) the effect in order to determine how to affect the gap reduction and how to measure your progress (or lack thereof). By adding to your efforts, you now begin to collect and analyze critical data that would affect your ability to determine your relative success or failure. For example, your process map becomes a value stream map, creating data boxes for each process step. Once the data have been collected, it is analyzed, and once again, you engage in root cause analyses. Having an understanding of the constraints and bottlenecks that might be causing the gap, you can effectively develop potential solutions.

In the majority of projects I have seen or in which I have participated, the team (or just one person!) comes up with several if not many possible solutions. Since most practices do not have unlimited resources, it is necessary to have a vetting process to cull the best potential solutions from the batch. This is often achieved using a priority matrix. Sometimes referred to as a Pugh matrix, this is a tool set that assigns a value to components of a possible solution and then ranks them based on a series of criteria, such as the resources required versus the expected benefits. The end goal is to find the one or two that, through consensus, will provide the greatest benefit with the least amount of risk and then graduate implementation to allow for observation and measurement of the results.

The tools in the Do phase include:

- Data Mining and Statistics;
- VSM;
- Brainstorming;
- Prioritization; and
- Hypothesis Testing.

Check (Study)

This phase defines the difference between PDCA and PDSA. In PDCA, the "C" stands for "check." In PDSA, the "S" stands for "study." For all intents and purposes, the two are quite interchangeable. The goal is to examine the change process and learn about the effects. You want to document what you observe both subjectively and quantitatively. In the Plan phase, you should have developed a system to measure the outcomes, and here is where that system is implemented. In any benefit/risk analysis, it goes without saying that you need to measure both the benefits and the risks, and it is not uncommon to find that implementation of a "fix" in one area "breaks" something in another area. For example, EMR technology is supposed to increase efficiency and reduce coding errors. In some studies, researchers found that while this may be true, there was an unexpected result of increased denials and down coding due to medical necessity problems. Another example is a practice that installed a television in the waiting room to reduce perceived waiting time but it had the unexpected effect of biasing continuing time estimates as patients would estimate waiting time based on the length of the program they were watching. I know of many practices that decided to outsource their billing function only to find that write-offs due to denials increased because the billing company used auto-posting systems that were not effective at catching payer payment errors.

It is here that you begin to compare metrics with goals. For example, maybe you reduced patient visit cycle time by three minutes instead of the seven minutes that was your goal. You can analyze the positive steps that resulted in the reduction while also analyzing what is preventing realization of the last four minutes. This type of analysis will help you to identify barriers and constraints that still exist, allowing you to attack those or, alternately, modify your goals if you are not able to make any further progress.

The tools used in the Check phase include:
- Control Charts;
- Data Checksheets and Worksheets;
- KPIs; and
- CTQ Trees.

Act

In the "Act" phase, the team comes back together to review the data collected in the prior step. By examining the data, the team determines the degree of success and/or failure and once again engages in brainstorming sessions to separate the things that worked from the things that didn't. This is a great time to tweak the recommended improvements. For example, you may want to define the time period prior to the visit that is most effective for having staff call patients to remind them to complete their intake paperwork. Or you may want to include a front-end scrubber as part of your A/R reduction plan in addition to other improvement steps. Most likely, by this point, you and the team will have received a wonderful education as to the process of the PDSA/PDCA and be able to define the knowledge and skills that were gained. The new process should be mapped and documented and made a part of the SOP.

Affected employees should be trained in the new process, and there should be a general buy-in regarding standardization and training. Now, hot off the trail of this project, the team should begin to plan for the next. Undoubtedly, during the Plan step, other issues and problems were identified that are next up in the queue of continuous improvement.

The tools in the Act phase include:
- Current Process and Future State Mapping;
- Process Standardization; and
- Formal Training.

Ramp Up Your PDSA Projects

Any PDSA begins with hunches, theories, and ideas. While I do not believe that intuition alone is a replacement for data and analysis, it can (and often does) point us in the right direction. In ramping up a project, we want to start with very small-scale tests and then move up to follow-up tests, a wider scale of tests, and then into the change phases. In our example of looking at ways to reduce wait time, we decided to focus on a small scale of drivers—namely, new patient intake packages. First, we timed three new Medicare patients and three new non-Medicare patients for one week to record the actual time it took each to complete the forms in the package and to determine if there was a difference between the two. The data gave us an average time of 22 minutes for Medicare patients and 17 minutes for non-Medicare patients. This prompted the team to add another short study to determine the reason for the difference. The team recorded the total number of questions asked by each patient group and what those questions were or to what they could be attributed. It turned out that the Medicare patients had a more difficult time reading some of the wording while the non-Medicare patients' questions were more focused on a particular paragraph in the financial responsibility form.

The goal of the team was to reduce new patient intake to 10 minutes—slightly longer than for established patients. To do this, from the results of the data collected, the team decided to do two things: one was to redesign the intake package, and the second was to figure out a way to get patients to complete the forms in advance of the appointment. This was a perfect opportunity to run a couple of different PDSA testing procedures simultaneously—one for the package design and one to reduce the intake time. The design team created three new designs for each patient type. For the Medicare patients, they first increased the type size to make it easier to read. They also simplified the package by removing duplicate and unnecessary forms. They timed six Medicare patients in a single day and found the time it took to complete the package was reduced by 9 minutes; from 22 to 13 minutes on average. For the non-Medicare group, the team studied the questions that were asked and concluded that a couple of paragraphs in the financial policy section were difficult to understand; they had been written by the practice's attorney and were not in lay terms. Consulting the attorney, the team reworded the paragraphs using more understandable terms and, likely by reducing the time involved in the questions being asked, reduced the average time to, surprisingly enough, 13 minutes—the same as the Medicare patients.

In the meantime, the second team mailed new patient packets to 10 new Medicare and 10 new non-Medicare patients that were due for their appointments during the next week. To their surprise, just over 50% showed up at the practice with their new patient packages complete (they estimated fewer than 10% would do this), shaving an incredible seven additional minutes from the average time it now took to intake a new patient.

This is all well and good but is not the end of the story. Remember, the Act phase of PDSA is to reexamine your goals and your gaps and to start again. The question came up regarding ways to improve the percentage of new patients that would complete the package in advance, and the process started over again.

PDSA Pitfalls

PDSA projects fail primarily due to three reasons. The first is making the goal too big, which ends up making the tests for the change too large too quickly. Remember, ramping means that you begin with a (very) small test and then increase it until you find the balance between action and planning. The second is not writing down the plan and documenting progress, successes, and failures, and/or failing to review what you do record with the team. PDSA is more than a process improvement platform; it is a learning device, and if the team doesn't take time to debrief both during and after the project, then the benefits of learning will be lost. The third mistake is not making a prediction of the outcomes. As stated above, we learn more by being surprised than by being correct. Make a guess as to what you expect to happen. Heck, let the team vote on who was closest without going over. If you don't have some expectation for an outcome, it makes is that much harder to assess how well you are learning as you go along.

IDEA

As if we haven't had enough acronyms, here comes another in the seemingly infinite vernacular of process improvement. IDEA stands for Investigate, Design, Execute, and Adjust. Similar to PDCA/PDSA, IDEA is a more rapid deployment platform and normally involves a less formal approach than some of the other platforms. IDEA is a bit more clear cut and has fewer tangential branches, and in many cases, does not follow the Team approach. While employing some of the same tools at the Deming wheel, IDEA is designed to address low-hanging fruit and more obvious "in your face" problems, eliminating the need for some of the data analysis steps. As with any process improvement project, I always recommend, at the least, the process in question is mapped. In fact, even processes NOT in question should be mapped as this is a great way to identify otherwise arcane problems for future projects.

Investigate, while similar to Plan, is normally less complex in its stages. Eliminating the team concept, this can usually be accomplished in a day or so or even in hours. Spend a day walking around the practice with a notepad and pen documenting every area of waste or possible error that you can find—redundancies, movement, organization, placement, delay, outdated references, poor technology, etc. Then, define the problems, give a brief background statement, pick the one that is most likely to bring the most benefit with the least risk, and determine the cause. This is a particularly good platform for process owners, and quite often, in a focused review, they know the problem and don't require a team approach to get to the core of the issue.

In the Design phase, you want to picture (or imagine, if you will) the idealized future state. In other words, you should ask yourself, "If I could redesign this from scratch (or do this over), I would . . ." This is not too far from a loose interpretation of reengineering without the massive disruption that often entails. Look at all possible solutions, and pick the best one.

Execute includes documenting the detailed goals of the project, outlining the steps (remember tactics, strategy, and logistics), and defining the expected outcome (including risks and potential collateral damage).

Finally, in the Adjust phase, the intent is to study the outcome and make changes (tweak) where necessary. While not formalized in this platform, it is always a good idea to, once the improved process is working and in place, create a process map and document the steps for training and compliance purposes.

FOCUS

Once again dipping into the acronym toolbox, we come out with a platform called FOCUS, which stands for:

- **F**ind a process improvement opportunity.
- **O**rganize an effort to work on improvement.
- **C**larify the current knowledge of the process.
- **U**ncover the root cause of the variation/waste/problem/poor outcome.
- **S**elect a strategy for improvement.

To keep from beating a dead horse, I am going to avoid the redundancies consistent among this and other platforms, instead, looking at the differences.

In the Find phase, you are looking from a higher level of review. For example, this might encompass an entire process or cycle, such as the billing cycle, recruiting and hiring new employees, or room turnaround time in an ambulatory surgery center or operating room, etc. Often, this platform is preferred by executives such as owners and administrators, originating from the reviews and analyses they conduct for the organization.

In the Organize phase, you may assign one or more staff members to work on the project, such as collecting pertinent data or developing a process map and someone to get involved in improving the process. In situations involving A/R, for example, this may include the coders or the data entry folks. Often times, those closest to the process in question are the key players in this type of rapid improvement model. In most cases, this does not involve a formal team effort, making this a bit more user-friendly in smaller organizations.

Clarifying the current knowledge of the process is another way of referring to the need to educate key players on the current state of the issue.

Uncovering the root cause remains one of the most important steps in the process improvement project, whether large or small, formal or informal. Without root cause analysis, you will rarely see any benefit from your efforts. In some situations, the cause will be clearly evident and won't require brainstorming sessions, while in other situations, it may be necessary to at least get a cross-disciplinary group of folks in the room to get some collaborative discussions going.

Selecting a strategy is where this platform can really diverge from the pattern we find in others in that it is not only acceptable but sometimes preferable to approach this from a less formal position. While the strategy may be as simple as developing an implementation plan, some folks use this step as a springboard to piggyback on a different platform, such as PDSA. While it may seem redundant, it actually is a more efficient way of coming up with dynamic solutions when high-level decisions are made regarding the need for a project.

As an example, I recently worked with a practice that wanted to look at the feasibility (from a standpoint of efficiency and profitability) of purchasing and installing an EMR system. In the interview process, I discovered that the health system that owned the physician group had mandated that the EMR be implemented, so an analysis of the effects became moot since it was going to happen regardless of the results. But it did not negate the importance of developing a process to implement, test, tweak, and analyze performance, which was the goal of the health system in the first place. In this case, we avoided much of the formality that would have been incurred to define and prioritize the project as it was already defined by the owners.

A3

A3 is a bit of a departure from some of the other deployment platforms we will study here. While A3 is still a force for process improvement, it focuses more on the process of problem solving than the formal process improvement models that are found in the other platforms. Most organizations effect what is known as "first-order" problems solving—that is, creating non-robust workarounds rather than real solutions to problems. Often, this type of approach creates potential collateral damage that may not be considered and therefore, appears unexpectedly and without contingency plans. A3 pushes toward the root cause of the problem. Without the root cause, the problem never really gets solved, only moved around within the cycle or the process. As with other process improvement platforms, root cause analysis is the fulcrum point for efficient and effective problem solving.

Ten Steps to A3 Success

A3 comprises 10 individual steps:

1. Conduct research to understand the current situation.
2. Conduct root cause analysis.
3. Devise countermeasures to address root causes.
4. Develop a target state.
5. Create an implementation plan.
6. Develop a follow-up plan with predicted outcomes.
7. Discuss plans with all affected parties.
8. Obtain approval for implementation.
9. Implement plans.
10. Evaluate the results.

As stated above, A3 is much more rooted in the area of problem solving and as such, tends to be front-heavy when cross-walking these steps to those of more common process improvement platforms, such as PDCA. For example, steps 1 to 8 of A3 are equivalent to the Plan step in PDCA (with step 5 planning the Do step and step 6 planning the Check step). Step 9 is the Do step, and step 10 is the Check step of PDCA. Based on the evaluation, another problem may be identified, and the A3 process starts again (Act).

Step 1: Understanding the Issues

Before any problem solving can begin, you must first have a firm grasp of the current situation, or what is often referred to as the "current state." This goes back to the idea of the Zen of process mapping, which is, "be the thing." Like other initial steps in process improvement, you begin with a process map. And while you don't necessarily go to the formal development of a value stream map, you do create data points for the steps in the process map. This idea is to quantify the potential problems that are the focus of this A3 event. For example, if you are looking to solve waiting time or cycle time issues, it requires the development of measurement systems to gather times for the different events. If you are looking at no-shows as a problem, you would want to calculate no-shows as a percentage of all scheduled visits or procedures and then quantify the reasons that patients didn't show up.

For example, if 8.4% of appointments turn into a no-show, and you find out that 61.7% of those occur because of transportation problems, you can begin to focus on solutions pertaining to the specific reasons for that problem. In one practice, we saw an increase in the number of patients that were showing up late for appointments. In a one-month study, we reported 17.2% of patients were late. When asked why they were late, nearly 70% said that being late meant they didn't have to wait as long to see the doctor. While that was mostly true for this group, it did have a rebound effect that resulted in pretty much everyone else having a longer wait time as schedules were adjusted for the late group. To fix this, we created a letter that explained to patients that if they were more than five minutes late, they would be shifted in the queue to behind the next patient in line, which could double their wait time. It was a very successful program that, without needing to go through a formal process improvement project, reduced late patients to just under 3.5%.

Step 2: Root Cause Analysis

Jumping right to the foundation of the problem (or problems), you engage root cause analysis tools, such as the fishbone diagram, to expedite your investigation of the causes for the problem(s). For example, a team trying to improve patient transport time recognized that the main problem was that patients were not arriving on time for their diagnostic procedures, causing severe backups in the diagnostic departments. The root cause analysis revealed that patients were arriving late because the hospital had no procedure for notifying appropriate personnel of a transportation need, and that transporters and RNs were not contacted directly by the requesting department.

Let's look at another common situation involving patients who show up late to the office for an appointment. One practice conducted a very good survey of late patients, asking one question: Why were you late?

Step 3: Develop Countermeasures

Countermeasures are the changes to be made to the work processes that will move the organization closer to ideal, or make the process more efficient, by addressing root causes. Documentation is quite important in this step, and you want to specify in writing the outcome, content, sequence, and task of work activities. The objective is to fix the problem—really fix the problem—rather than creating a workaround, which is always temporary and often creates collateral issues. Countermeasures sometimes involve contingency plans, which are used to counteract or respond to situations that may not always be avoidable.

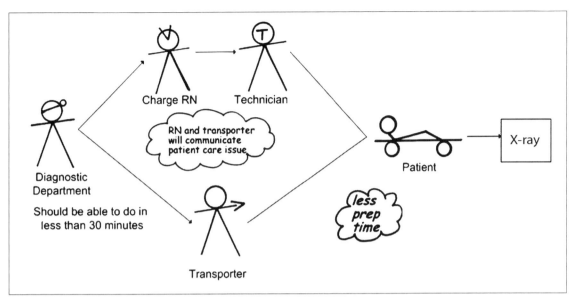

FIGURE 47. A story-board example of an A3 Project.[a]

For example, denials are a reality when you submit claims to third-party payers. You can't avoid denials but you can have a contingency plan on how to deal with them when they arrive. The idea is to mitigate the damage. Another example is dealing with patients who have a language barrier. Some states require that the practice use an interpreter at its own cost so having a contingency plan allows you to move forward with the least negative impact. Countermeasures may be as simple as a written policy, such as financial policies, or as complex as building a model, such as with disaster planning.

Step 4: Develop a Target State

In this step, the specific countermeasure or contingency plan should be recorded, and the expected improvement or mitigation should be projected using quantifiable metrics. One example is developing a new target for restructuring the way in which patients scheduled for MRIs are processed to reduce the time between studies. In one study involving patient transport time, the target condition for a revamped patient transportation process was sketched out, as illustrated in Figure 47.

---

[a] *This example comes from a collaborative research project between Community Medical Center of Missoula, Montana, and Montana State University in Bozeman. Dr. Durwood Sobek, Montana State University, Principal Investigator; Cindy Jimmerson, Community Medical Center, Co-principal Investigator; Manimay Ghosh, Montana State University, Graduate Research Assistant.*

Step 5: The Implementation Plan

The implementation plan should be a detailed list that includes the actions needed in order to get the countermeasures in place and realize the target condition. It should also include the name of the individual(s) responsible for each task and a due date. The latter is a critical element as it allows you to estimate the resources required for the tasks. It should also include other relevant items, such as cost, target dates, time lines and requirements, constraints, risks, etc.

For example, if you are working through an HR problem, such as excessive time required to fill a position, and you have already gained an understanding of the reasons for the problem (root cause), the plan might outline a new system to define, post, review, and vet the applicants prior to the interview process and maybe even eliminate one layer in that process itself. The plan might include items related to exactly what steps would need to take place to reduce the total time to, say, two weeks. It would set a target date for when the improvement would be done. It might include any costs or even cost savings, such as a reduced cycle time. You might include constraints, such as advertising lead time or personnel availability to review online responses from Internet job sites. The reason for the implementation plan is twofold; it helps to keep the people involved motivated, and it prevents process drift, the condition that occurs when tangential paths begin to take focus over the primary process itself.

For example, while exploring the viability of using Internet-based job sites, you come across an ad for HR systems designed to streamline the job-search process. While this may be relevant to your organization, it is outside the scope of the project. If it is important, it should be evaluated separately as a possible option or even a new project, but because it is not part of the original project, either the project plan should be reevaluated, a parallel investigation could take place, or it should be put on hold until after the original project is complete.

Step 6: The Follow-up Plan

Remember, A3 is a problem-solving model, and in order for it to be successful, the people involved should know (or be effectively learning) how to solve problems. The follow-up step fulfills two primary purposes; the first is to see whether the solution worked and second, actually related to the first, is to see how well the A3 team learned this particular skill. Many a project goes untested, and as a result, one never knows if the solution really worked. Anecdotally, we often talk about the successes or failures based on a remark, compliment, or complaint here or there. Without a structured system to measure the results, we really won't know if it worked or, perhaps more importantly, how well it worked.

For example, let's say you set out to solve a problem about complaints over waiting time. One solution is to put a television in the waiting room to divert patients' attention from waiting. As a result, the complaints stopped or lessened. Did you solve your problem? Well, what was your goal? If it was to reduce complaints, maybe; but if you don't conduct a patient satisfaction study that is random and similar both before and after, you really don't know. If the goal was to improve patient cycle time to increase efficiency and the number of patients seen on a given day, then how would you know without a follow-up study? The answer, of course, is that you would not. The follow-up plan is a critical step in the problem solving to ensure the implementation plan was executed, the target condition (goal) realized, and the expected results achieved. Remember, for this to occur, you must have first defined your target state, which, for all intents and purposes, is what you use to define success.

It is important to note that you are evaluating two things here: the implementation plan itself and the outcome of the solution. Let's build on our example of waiting time. The A3 project manager sets the waiting time goal (target state) at a maximum of 30 minutes. Each day, five days a week for four weeks, four patients are selected at random, and their waiting time is measured. This goes on for three months to identify the variability (if any) from the target state and actual time. After that time, a determination will be made as to the relative success of the solution. In addition, the plan will be reviewed by the A3 team members to identify the variability from their different target states: was the project completed on time and within cost expectations? Were any of the risks realized, such as any collateral issues like patient complaints regarding what shows were on the TV, which was installed to reduce the patients' perception of wait time; arrangement of seating to access the TV screen; whether the TV was too loud or not loud enough, etc.

Finally, this information will be discussed with the team to evaluate the effectiveness of not just the project, but how well the team learned problem-solving skills.

Step 7: Communicate the Plan

In many cases, the people who approve of or fund the projects are not directly involved in the development and/or execution phases. Therefore, it is very important to communicate the plan to those folks if we expect to get the green light, especially if there is the need for additional resources. In addition, by keeping the decision makers in the loop, the team can evoke a kind of "post-close" perception that creates a higher level of confidence in the team. To achieve the greatest level of success in this step, it is recommended that the type of communication occurs at every critical juncture and sentinel event, not just the final plan.

In an example involving prescription refills, let's say there is a problem involving pulling the wrong chart when the last name of the patient is the same as the last name of another (or several other) patient(s). The A3 team leader weighs the evidence and determines that there is a need to change the hand-off sequence for charts being pulled such that a second person documents that he or she has checked some other data other than just the patient's last name. To accomplish this, it requires that someone from a different department (maybe a clinical person in addition to an administrative person) will be required to participate. Once this target solution (or countermeasure) has been decided upon, the A3 team leader will meet with key players in that department to solicit their concurrence and cooperation and to work together to implement the changes.

Step 8: Obtain Approval (or Show Me the Money!)

The purpose of step 8 is get authorization to invoke the plan (solution, countermeasure, process change, etc.). And authorization often includes approval of the required resources. This can include time, money, personnel, risk, or even physical space. When the authorizer, as it were, and the A3 team leader or champion are different people, this can be a more difficult step. There is a big difference between knowing enough to buy something and enough to sell it. The team leader should, by this time, know enough about the project to sell it, but he or she is selling it to someone who, perhaps, has little or no knowledge of the work and effort that has gone into the learning process. This is precisely why step 7 is so important; regular and consistent communication keeps everyone at least on the same page and prevents the need to "start from scratch" every time an approval is required. For this step to be successful, the authorizer needs to be on board with the proposal.

In our prior example (problem with pulling the wrong chart for a prescription refill), the A3 team leader is in the position to approve the hand-off from the medical records person since he or she is in the same department but not from the clinical department head. If there was a lack of communication or a communication breakdown between this person and the clinical department manager, it could result in an implementation delay due to all the reasons we know exist, such as politics, policies, egos, etc. The delay would be magnified if, for example, in order for the policy to be changed, the administrator required approval from both department managers.

Step 9: Implementation

Implementation begins with testing the solutions. Hopefully, in step 5 (development of the implementation plan), these systems were defined, including who would be responsible, how the testing would occur, what would be measured, and when it would take place. One practice identified a problem regarding the extended time it took patients to complete the new-patient intake package. For those patients that did not show up early enough before their appointment to complete the package, the physician had to wait for them to finish up and be escorted to the exam room. Reality check: for every minute a physician spends waiting for a patient, revenue is lost.

Two solutions were agreed to during the vetting process: streamline the package by removing unnecessary forms and rewording areas where it was noted that a significant number of questions were asked by new patients. The former was more oriented toward the staff—ensuring that the minimum number of forms were included to allow for an accurate clinical assessment and compliance with all applicable laws, rules, and regulations. The latter, however, was dependent upon feedback from the patients, and both of these solutions, when combined, netted the result of reducing the amount of time required to complete the package to the desired goal. To test the latter solution, the practice had tallied all of the questions asked by patients concerning the intake forms over the past month, placing them into five different buckets (i.e., unable to understand, not applicable to their situation, difficult to read, etc.). Then the practice introduced three different versions of the intake package and tracked the number of questions that were asked in those same five buckets. Two things occurred; first, the practice was able to identify which packet resulted in the greatest reduction of questions; and secondly, it enabled the practice to make a few more tweaks that reduced the time even more.

Step 10: Evaluate the Result(s)

Step 10 ties back to step 6 (the follow-up plan). There, you commit to writing how and when the results would be tracked and measured to better understand the variance of the results from your goals and/or predictions. If the actual results differ from the predicted ones, research needs to be conducted to figure out why, modify the process, and repeat implementation and follow-up until the goal is met or it is accepted that the goal cannot, in fact, be achieved. The latter may necessitate a redefining of the goal, or if the goal is mission critical and cannot be changed (i.e., due to laws and/or licensing regulations), a different and more robust platform may need to be employed.

Let's say that you attacked a particular problem involving turnaround time for an imaging procedure with a goal to turn the room around and have it ready for the next patient within 15 minutes—a reduction of 10 minutes over your current time. Several steps were instituted, including using anti-microbial-treated table paper (saves time in cleaning the table between visits) and preparing the IV infusion mechanisms ahead so that, as one patient was being scanned, the setup for the next patient was being prepared. The person assigned in the follow-up plan to conduct the study takes five random measurements every day for 10 days during the month and then computes the averages of each of those days, as follows:

- Day 1—14 minutes
- Day 2—16 minutes
- Day 3—11 minutes
- Day 4—14 minutes
- Day 5—15 minutes
- Day 6—23 minutes
- Day 7—13 minutes
- Day 8—12 minutes
- Day 9—14 minutes
- Day 10—11 minutes

The results are shown in Figure 48.

Note that both the mean and the median were under 15 minutes (14.5 and 14, respectively) so it can be concluded that the goal was met. But notice that on day 6, the average was 23 minutes—statistically speaking, an outlier. Part of the evaluation step includes looking at outliers to see why they occurred. In this case, the person responsible for preparing the IVs in advance failed to obtain enough IV poles, so the IVs could not be prepared in advance, adding nearly nine minutes to the total time.

Summary

As noted above, A3 is a very focused deployment platform that is primarily used to solve well-defined problems where a more formal deployment plan might prove to be cumbersome and inefficient. A3 projects are very good at helping people to develop problem-solving skills as it follows a very logical and efficient step-wise process.

KAIZEN

I have saved the section on Kaizen for last; not because it is least important but because it is a different concept that is sometimes seen as a deployment platform and other times in-

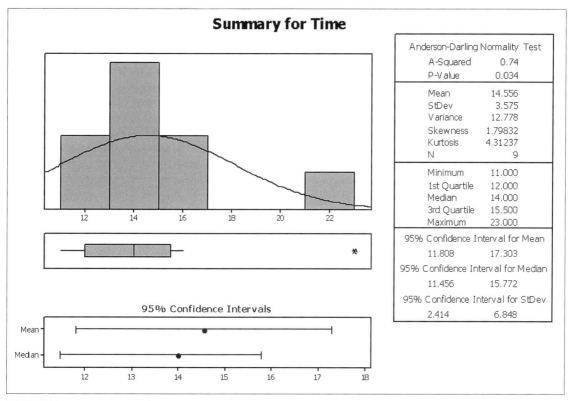

FIGURE 48. **Summary for time.**

corporates deployment platforms in its process. Realistically, a discussion of Kaizen could fill an entire chapter or, more likely, an entire book. The following attempts to lay out the basic concepts of Kaizen in a way that will assist you with understanding its importance, objectives, and process.

Kaizen comes from two Japanese words: "Kai," meaning change, and "Zen," meaning good or for the better. Kaizen is a concept designed to produce continuous small changes such that, over time, as each small improvement builds on the other, the final result is a model that creates a culture of overall and larger scale improvements. Like PDSA, Kaizen is designed to address focused issues or problem areas; but unlike PDSA, Kaizen follows more of a timed than a pragmatic approach. And while it is structured, it is structured as a model and not a process. This means that it is, in essence, a shell that holds the process that provides the opportunity for improvement. This is why Kaizen will often employ other deployment platforms, such as DMAIC or PDSA.

In Western parlance, Kaizen has become more of a rapid-response methodology and is often seen as a type of a "blitz" improvement process. By implication, Kaizen events are seen as rapid and therefore consuming a short period of time; most often resulting in an event that lasts no longer than five days. This idea of has taken on a life of its own in that when most folks nowadays talk about Kaizen events, they are mostly saying a five-day event. This idea, unfortunately, has resulted in many a project that has had negative or poor results; not because a Kaizen event can't be conducted in five days (or sometimes less) but rather because many people don't consider that Kaizen has two parts: preparation and execution.

When most of the Lean Six Sigma people I meet discuss the "five-day Kaizen," they are referring to the execution part without considering the preparation aspect. The latter is actually what takes the most time and, in reality, can add four- or five-fold to the total time committed to the actual Kaizen event (execution).

Now, some will argue this point, believing that preparation is separate and not part of the Kaizen event itself, and I welcome their thoughts and ideas. My experience, however, has been that, without a thorough preparation, Kaizen is nothing more than an extended brainstorming session. At best, it may likely produce good ideas and solutions suitable for testing. At worst, it can prove a total waste of time and resources, turning an organization away from ever trying it again in the future.

Before we continue, it is important to remember that a Kaizen event is part and parcel of a Lean project even though it can be used as a freestanding model. Kaizen events are often used to kick-off a more involved Lean project, and as such, start out in response to specific functional issues rather than originating from data drivers. As such, while process mapping is an integral part of the event, VSM will become more important as one of the goals is to convert the functional issues into data-drivers.

As with other Lean and Six Sigma process improvement projects, Kaizen events respond best to team development. Unlike larger or more complex platforms, teams are often informal, even though they assume some formal organizational elements. For example, it is still important to have a team leader, subject experts, process owners, etc. And unless the team is larger (more than 10 people) or involves ad hoc and/or outside members, it is normally not necessary to have a separate facilitator. As with other aspects of process improvement projects, communication with stakeholders and upper management is critical. Also, defining roles and responsibilities for team members is just as necessary here as with larger projects.

In my experience, there are six characteristics of an effective Kaizen event:
1. The project has been selected.
2. Resources are dedicated and defined prior to starting.
3. As much data as possible are collected prior to initial meeting.

4. The team works full time on the event/project.
5. Implementation of recommendations is made immediately.
6. Resources are made available by upper management to complete the improvement process.

Preparation

Some Kaizen events will involve the development of a charter, similar to what we saw with the DMAIC platform, although it is usually less complex and does not delineate all of the components. As a Kaizen event is often a part of the DMAIC platform, the charter may simply be a subset of the DMAIC charter. The workhorse of a Kaizen event is the VSM. If you already read about VSM in the previous chapter, then it is easy to understand how the preparation phase of the Kaizen event may be quite time consuming. Remember, before you get to the VSM, you first need the process map. Then it is necessary to complete the data box for each step, which will likely include data mining, statistical analysis, measurement systems analysis, and other tools to ensure that the data are appropriate, accurate, timely, and above all, useful. Most Kaizen events will *not* focus on the entire VSM but rather on one particular step or section of the map; hence the idea of being able to "blitz" through in five days or less.

For example, in reviewing patient visit cycle time, you may have identified many different steps organized into several sections, such as check-in, provider visit, diagnostic studies, treatments, check-out, etc. It would be completely appropriate to conduct a Kaizen event for each of those sections. Again, you might take the check-in component, which consists of several different steps and commit a Kaizen event just for that component. And in the process, you may employ multiple PDSA episodes to deal with the different details involved in one or more steps in that component.

Preparation also involves team development. If this is a new team, there will be a period that involves the usual team development dynamics (see Chapter 3) before it becomes effective. Preparation also involves scheduling and resource allocation for meetings, including locations, times, dates, etc. This is particularly time consuming if the event will include ad hoc members and/or outside experts.

Execution

As you can now understand, preparing for a Kaizen event can take weeks, and it is not unusual for this to sometimes extend to months, particularly when there is a need to engage in design of experiments to obtain real-time data, such as with cycle times or clinical investigations. Day zero of a Kaizen event is often a meeting of the key players, including stakeholders, to verify that everything is in place and ready to go. Nothing is more discouraging than to have the first day of a Kaizen event fall apart due to lack of preparation.

Hopefully, if the preparation went well, you will have a meeting place that facilitates the efficiency that is required for a Kaizen event. Some organizations already have a "war room" of sorts that is used for meetings, educational events, conferences, and training. Being self-contained is important in that the room has everything needed without having to switch rooms. This might include audio/visual equipment, Internet access, telephones, white boards, etc. In some cases, it is better to have the meeting off-site to exclude the potential for other employees to interrupt with messages and questions for participants. In effect, I like to observe the "100 mile" rule. This means that participants are interrupted for issues that would come up if they were 100 miles or more from the office.

A tough rule to enforce is no cell phones, e-mail, or text messaging. Sometimes during the event itself, it may be necessary to contact a subject expert or other process owner (not on the team) to clarify a point or validate data; this is not what I am talking about. If you have been in any meetings or conferences over the past couple of years, you probably know what I am referring to. Any outside communication needs to be relevant to the topic at hand and cannot include the normal texting communications that most of us experience on a day-to-day basis. I could go on with specific examples, but the point is, participants need to be focused. If you don't control for these types of distractions, you can expect to waste a lot of time during the event. Think about it; if someone can be absent on the phone during the event without a negative impact, then maybe that person shouldn't be on the team. If the person's role is critical (which every team member's role should be), then the individual needs to be present and focused the entire time.

The other rule that seems to be very effective for Kaizen events is to have food available. I'm not sure what it is, but my experience is that pretty much every meeting is more successful if refreshments are provided for participants.

While a Kaizen event can be any amount of time, we typically conduct them in anywhere from three to five days. Some include a prep week that ends after the first day of the event and then continues the following four days with a DMAIC model. For example, during the prep week, stakeholders and the team leader develop the objective for the event. Participants are chosen, and the team is assembled for a full day of training on process improvement in general and Kaizen specifically. Process and value stream mapping projects are completed (or at least drafted), and preliminary data are defined and collected. Finally, a logistics plan is developed that defines how the event will be conducted (includes the "where," "when," and "who" components).

Beginning with day one (let's call it Monday), the process map, value stream map, and data are reviewed, analyzed, and summarized. Day two (and sometimes part of day three) involves brainstorming sessions for cause-and-effect work. The idea here is to identify the root cause of the waste within the process or the problems that were discovered. During this phase, it is also important to continue brainstorming to find possible solutions. Day three (and sometimes part of day four) is committed creating an action list of possible solutions from the suggestions that have been made. This would include prioritization techniques and testing solutions, at least theoretically. When the best of the best have been identified and tests meet expectations, an implementation plan and methods to train employees are developed. The rest of day four and day five involve documenting results and presenting to upper management and/or stakeholders.

More often than not, the end of the event is not the end of the project but rather the beginning of the implementation of the solutions. To do this, you may find that you require additional resources, and without approval from the stakeholders, it is pretty much impossible to obtain. And don't forget to develop a follow-up plan, complete with the "who," "how," "when," and "what" components of the plan. Figure 49 is a diagram of what this type of Kaizen plan might look like.

I also would like to discuss a typical (if there is such a thing) five-day event to demonstrate the steps that take place and the outcomes we might expect. Here, we might see the following schedule:

Day One

On day one, we pull together the team of process owners and experts and conduct training, often using examples specific to the organization. This get's everyone on the same page and introduces how the Kaizen event will be conducted as it relates to specific issues, rules, politics, etc.

Day Two

On day two, the process maps and value stream maps are developed. In order for this to work, preparatory work must have been done to collect the data that will be required (e.g., denial rates, wait time, A/R, visits per period, etc). These data are then compiled into the VSM. It is now that the specific VSM steps will be reviewed to decide which ones will be addressed during the event, if this decision was not already made by management.

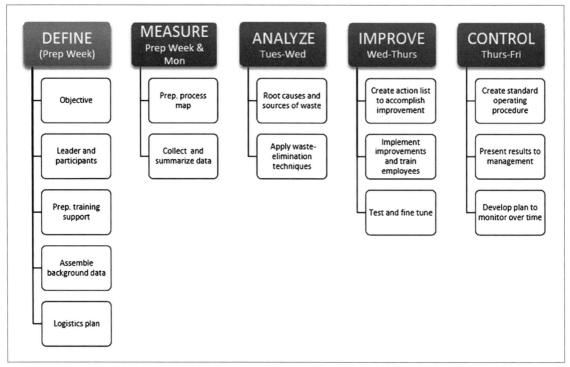

FIGURE 49.   Prep-week concept of a Kaizen event.

Day Three

On day three, the team spends the day on cause-and-effect relationships, researching the validity of those reasons, identifying root causes, and creating suggestions for solutions.

Day Four

Day four is committed to finalizing solutions based on the prior day's root causes identification. This includes vetting those solutions using a prioritization matrix. When the solution (or solutions) that appear to be the best of the best have been identified, they are tested.

This can often be a confusing stage of the process for some people because they associate testing at this point to the type of testing that is conducted following implementation of a new or fixed process step, and it is not. When we talk about testing during a Kaizen event, we are referring to a type of brainstorming session during which process owners and subject experts are asked to map through the changes and identify potential failure points that might occur from the change. If substantive problems are discovered, it usually results in either fixing the solution or abandoning it in favor of the next on the list.

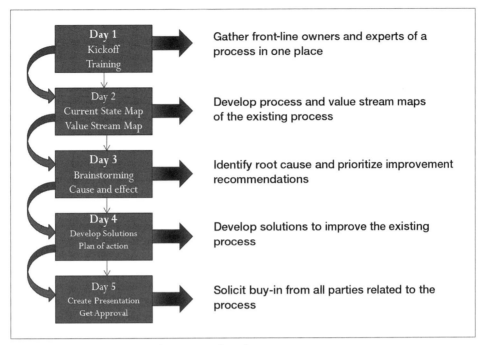

FIGURE 50. Summary of steps in a five-day Kaizen event.

Day Five

As discussed in the prior event type, final implementation will normally require some type of approval from upper management, even if it doesn't involve additional resources. Critical information here involves benefit/risk analyses, ROI (if that is required), integration planning. and a follow-up plan to validate the results of implementation.

Figure 50 is an illustration of what this type of Kaizen event might look like.

No matter what type of Kaizen event is implemented and irrespective of the amount of time it takes to complete, there are certain criteria necessary to make it work. I already mentioned the need for a dedicated room, focused participants, and food. Here are some others:

- The room should have lots of wall space since these types of projects use a lot of writing pads and sticky notes.
- There should be an agenda for each day, and the day should start on time and end on time.
- Confidentiality is a must, particularly regarding individual discussions. The best way to destroy any team event is to compromise trust among the participants.

- Progress (or lack of it) should be communicated regularly to the stakeholders. This is primarily the responsibility of the team leader.
- Regular feedback and even interviews should be conducted with team members to ensure that there aren't any hidden conflicts among participants.

As a final outcomes measurement, a survey should be sent to participants 30 days after the event to get final feedback and elicit ideas to improve these types of activities in the future. Remember, like every other aspect of process improvement, the Kaizen event is a learning experience designed to build a culture of process improvement within the organization.

SEVEN

What's Next:
According to Frank

WOW! That's the best word I can think of to describe my view of our industry right now. As of the writing of this book, we in healthcare are facing perhaps the most dynamic potential for change in our history. Barack Obama won, according to many pundits, by a landslide in a campaign that reflected voters' need for something different.

Today is Sunday, August 16, 2009, and congress went on its summer recess without having a healthcare bill ready for the President to sign as initially projected during his campaign. During the last two weeks, town hall meetings have sprung up around the county; and whether contrived or not, have been spirited, to say the least, representing passionate responses from those on both sides of the fence (as well as those in the middle). The big question on both mainstream and cable news programs, as well as the hundreds of political blogs out there, is whether there will be a new healthcare bill signed before the end of 2009, and more importantly, what it will look like. AARP, once on board with the President's plan and then not, spring-boarded a substantial controversy, especially among the elderly population. And who has a clue anymore what is information compared with what is misinformation. The President says he has no intention of creating a single-payer system while his opponents say that is exactly what he is proposing. The Congressional Budget Office disagrees sharply with the administration's projection of the cost of the plan (saying it will cost significantly more), fueling concerns over who is going to pay for this plan. And the most incredible thing is that all of this is happening before we even have a plan!

From what I can decipher from all of the conflicting information is that there are currently either three or five proposals; and somewhere along the way, the "gang of six" is going to merge them into something that everyone in the House and Senate can agree upon. Yet no one can say whether the American people will agree, as well. Some people report that in order to pay to insure the currently uninsured, we will have to take $500 billion from Medicare. Imagine how that went over with the over-65 population! Others say that is simply not true. And you and I are left to decide who (or whom) is telling the truth and who, if anyone, is lying.

Simply stated, these are exciting times we are living in! Personally, I am overloaded with information, and whether it becomes a single payer, multiple payer, no payer, or whatever, the fact is there are going to be significant changes in the near future. It seems like the only thing that everyone (except maybe the private payers right now) can agree upon is that something does need to change; that if we continue the way we are going, the entire healthcare system will be broke. Who knows!

I have my own idea of what solutions might work but no one in the government has called me to ask my opinion. How about tort reform? Well, there go the trial lawyers. How about we just hold the insurance companies accountable under current rules, regulations, and laws? Is it me, or does it feel like the only ones that have to abide by HIPAA are physicians, hospitals, and patients, and not the insurance companies? Maybe if they were just included in the Sherman anti-trust laws, as are physicians and other healthcare providers, that would close a very expensive loophole in the law. Maybe all we need is a large enough group of legislators that are willing to stand up to the insurance industry and hold it accountable to do the right thing; that is, a group that isn't influenced by the huge amount of money spent by health insurers to support their campaigns.

How about the cost of drugs in this country? Why can't we purchase drugs directly from Canada or Mexico? On that note, why can't Medicare negotiate directly with the drug makers for better prices? Sheesh! I know, let's allow physicians to collectively bargain like other professionals. How about strike rights?

OK. So maybe I have more questions than suggestions but why aren't these questions being asked; and if they are, why aren't they being answered or addressed? Whoops, another question . . . I heard a commentator today make a statement that physicians are responsible for the largest share of healthcare expenditures, and he said that as though it was a fact yet nothing could be further from the truth. Depending on the source you consult, physicians consume less than a third of all healthcare dollars spent in this country.

What the heck. While we're in the neighborhood, let's look at other significant changes looming in the immediate future. I just read that consulting codes will no longer be included in CPT 2010. I guess that's good news but it creates another layer of major change that providers will have to adjust to within only a relatively short period of time.

How about ICD-10? We can't even effectively handle the 14,000 or so CPT and HCPCS codes in the system now. How in the heck are we going to integrate some 88,000 new codes and expect to survive? I know, other countries have done this without a hitch but not according to the physicians and office managers I have interviewed from those countries. One study estimates that the cost of implementation of ICD-10 will be anywhere between $83,290 for a small practice to $2.7 million for a large practice.[1]

For those that believe that technology is the solution to what ails us, just take a look at electronic medical records (EMRs). Sure, they work in some cases but I have witnessed more than my share of practices that have been decimated by implementation (or attempted implementation) of EMR systems. My dad used to tell me that it's OK to be lucky when you're lucky, but not only is an EMR system not the solution to many problems practices face, it actually creates problems for some that didn't have problems before. President Bush announced his goal that every American would have an EMR in the near future, and for his part, President Obama has continued to promote this goal. For this to happen, every medical practice will need to implement an EMR system. And for this to happen, the benefit of such a system has to outweigh the risks or how can medical practices be expected to open their doors to this technology?

Without getting into citing them all, I have read dozens and dozens of articles and studies (as well as conducted my own) that conflict on whether EMR systems are really more efficient or add to quality outcomes. Nearly all of them, however, do talk about possible ways to improve the overall financial and quality benefits of EMR systems, yet I wonder if the vendors are listening.

Speaking of vendors, here is another constraint to practice efficiency that I hope to see improved in the future. From my count, there are perhaps nearly 1500 different practice management systems (PMSs) out there, and they come in every size, shape, and form. But mostly they have disparate database models that prohibit the effective collection and sharing of critical data. And the feds are not exempt from this. Accessing public information files that contain enough information to make the data valuable is nearly a full-time job and requires that the person who wants the data be some kind of expert in data mining and analysis.

Go to any Medical Group Management Association conference and look at the vendors; the majority represent some form of emerging technology, and many of those propose data solutions for practices. Again, while a step in the right direction, much of the value of these systems depends on the ability to pull accurate information from the practice, which, in turn, depends on the current PMS. As a data analyst, I marvel at how much time it takes to enter all of that valuable information into the software and then how incredibly difficult it is to get it back out in some usable format. And have you ever been involved in trying to transition from one PMS to another? I have, and my experience is that it is a nightmare. One physician told me it was akin to having an autopsy without the benefit of death! Once your best friend, when you decide to go with another vendor, you are pretty much on your own when it comes to migrating your data from the old to the new system. We don't need a single-payer system, we need a single-standard system; one that is polymorphic such that it can be fully transportable.

Stark is another area of continual consternation for physician practices (as well as hospitals and now pharmaceutical companies). The laws are so complex that I refer to the entire Stark world as the consultants' and lawyers' employment act of 2005. Actually, if you look at the entire scope of the overregulated world in which a physician operates, it is easy to see why so many physicians are considering walking away from the practice of medicine. What other small businesses can do, physician practices cannot do. I grant that there are those who would, in the absence of some form of regulation, take advantage of loopholes, but the degree of complexity moves this from the sublime to the ridiculous.

I have, in the past several years, worked as an expert in the capacity of litigation support representing physicians in nearly every stage of civil and criminal problems, from repayment demands to indictments involving fraud and abuse, and nearly all of them have one thing in common: the complexity of the rules and regulations. For example, there are three studies that conclude that the rate of disagreement on the level of E/M codes is around the 50% mark irrespective whether the person coding the event is a physician or a professional certified coder with many years of experience.[2-4] Most recently, I was involved in a case in which the physicians were under investigation based almost exclusively on their fees for a group of procedures, even though there isn't a single line of standing legislation that mandates the methodology a physician must use in order to establish charges or just how much a physician may or may not charge for a given procedure or service.

Medical malpractice is also looming as another constraint physicians face with regard to the need to practice defensive medicine. In some cases, the insurance costs have increased so dramatically that physicians have chosen to abandon coverage altogether, advising patients in advance that, should they choose to come after the physician with a claim of malpractice, their ability to collect huge damages may be severely limited. In my state of Florida, it doesn't seem that this has done much to limit their patient volume. In fact, more practices than ever are also choosing to dump payers altogether, instead practicing a form of free enterprise not often seen in our industry. Gruber et al.[5] have shown conclusively, at least in my opinion, that physicians are becoming more profitable treating uninsured patients as opposed to insured patients and for no other reason than payers have so deeply discounted their payments that it is just not reasonable to assume that they can any longer afford to operate under these financial constraints.

And the list goes on but here is the most incredible concept to me, and this is the world according to Frank: If you are armed with the tools and techniques that are discussed in this book, it doesn't matter what happens! Think about it. Whether we end up with government-controlled healthcare or the private payers continue to underpay physicians; whether we have ICD-10 or not; and whether it gets to a point where no physician can afford malpractice insurance or whether the majority of practices simply stop taking insurance altogether, those who have built a model of process improvement based on the tools and techniques discussed in this book will thrive. Not because this is the final and ultimate compendium of Lean and Six Sigma for medical practices and certainly not because I am a guru of process improvement, but rather because, in the simplest of terms, they work. Working from a successful model all but guarantees that, no matter what the landscape looks like, you will be able to navigate your way to the most efficient and profitable state in which you can exist. Really!

Depending on who you are and what you do for a living, how these changes will likely affect you will be different. Physicians will still be held culpable for the final outcome of the encounter or event; and therefore, perhaps they, more than anyone else, need to take this as seriously as possible. Not only do docs have the most to gain, they have the most to lose. Medical staff will require additional training and education in order to adapt to rapid changes. Vendors will need to be more end-user oriented and not just design a system based on what they think the end user needs or wants. This will work only if and when the vendors use several of the tools discussed in this book to "become the customer." If you are a healthcare consultant, you better take the shift from functional to analytical seriously because it is beginning to dominate the decision structure of many practices and other healthcare organizations. Things change, and if consultants don't move to the front edge of change, the value of their services will decline precipitously. Payers need to realize that we (the provider side, the general healthcare consumer, and business owners) are at the end of our rope with regards to the games they play to build profits on the backs of healthcare providers and subscribers. Based on the latest National Health Insurer Report Card published by the American Medical Association, payers pay nothing in one out of five claims; and in one out of four that they do pay, they pay incorrectly or inaccurately. In fact, I would venture to opine that the payers have more control over the cost of healthcare than any other entity, and if all they did were to incorporate some process improvement projects, they could contribute significantly to lowering the overall cost of healthcare. It's amazing how far a little transparency will go.

Finally, we need our legislators to legislate and our enforcers to enforce. As with other areas of concern, we don't need more laws, we simply need someone to stand up and enforce those on the books. One standard equally applied with a little process improvement thrown in, and maybe we can have a healthcare industry rather than a healthcare crisis.

References

1. *The Impact of Implementing ICD -10.* Nachimson Advisors, LLC; October, 2008.
2. King MS, Sharp L, Lipsky MS. Accuracy of CPT evaluation and management coding by family physicians. *J Am Board Fam Pract.* 2001;14:184-192.
3. Kikano GE, Goodwin MA, Stange KC. A comparison of medical record documentation with actual billing in community family practice. *Arch Fam Med.* 2000;9:68-71.
4. King MS, Lipsky MS, Sharp L. Expert agreement in Current Procedural Terminology, evaluation and management coding. *Arch Intern Med.* 2002;162:316-320.
5. Gruber J, Rodriguez D. How much uncompensated care do doctors provide? *Journal of Health Economics.* 2007;26:1151–1169.

INDEX